Living with Tourette Syndrome

"Wonderfully compassionate, and comprehensive . . . This book will serve for many years . . . for all families with Tourette Syndrome."

> — *Sue Levi-Pearl, Liaison, Medical and Scientific Programs, Tourette Syndrome Association, Inc.*

Depression: What Families Should Know

"It's clear, authoritative, sensitive—an easy read about a heavy subject."

> — *Sol Gordon, Ph.D., Professor Emeritus, Syracuse University*

"A valuable resource to the most hidden victims of depression—the loved ones of the sufferer."

> — *Melvin Sabshin, M.D., Medical Director, The American Psychiatric Association*

How to Get Out of the Hospital Alive

"It is important to your survival to be informed, and this book is an important reference."

> — *Bernie S. Siegel, M.D., author of* Love, Medicine and Miracles

Strokes: What Families Should Know

"An excellent source of information. It is written with a great sensitivity and understanding of the problems of stroke patients and their families."

> — *Bruce B. Grynbaum, M.D., P.C., Rusk Institute of Rehabilitation Medicine, New York University Medical Center*

Coping with Chronic
HEARTBURN

**What You Need to Know About
Acid Reflux and GERD**

Elaine Fantle Shimberg

St. Martin's Paperbacks

COPING WITH CHRONIC HEARTBURN

Copyright © 2001 by Elaine Fantle Shimberg.

All rights reserved. No part of this book may be used or reproduced in any manner whatsoever without written permission except in the case of brief quotations embodied in critical articles or reviews. For information address St. Martin's Press, 175 Fifth Avenue, New York, NY 10010.

Library of Congress Catalog Card Number: 00–045998

ISBN: 0-312-98206-2
EAN: 80312-98206-5

Printed in the United States of America

St. Martin's Griffin edition / February 2001
St. Martin's Paperbacks edition / April 2002

St. Martin's Paperbacks are published by St. Martin's Press, 175 Fifth Avenue, New York, NY 10010.

10 9 8 7 6 5 4

Dedicated to the memory of
Marty Weill

Author's Note

The information contained in this book reflects the author's research and is intended to help you better understand heartburn, gastroesophageal reflux disease, and its various effects on individuals. It is in no way intended to replace advice by a qualified medical professional. Medical opinions specific to you can be given only by a physician who has examined you and is aware of your unique medical history.

Never self-diagnose. Always seek help from a qualified physician.

Contents

Chapter One

What Is Gastroesophageal Reflux Disease? • How the Digestive System Works • What Causes Gastroesophageal Reflux? • How Is Gastroesophageal Reflux Disease Diagnosed?

Chapter Two

Are You Under Chronic Stress? • Are You Pregnant? • Are You Over Age Fifty? • Are You Overweight? • Infants and Children Can Have GERD • Do You Have Asthma? • Does Your Job Require Heavy Lifting, Stooping, or Squatting? • Do You Have a Hiatal Hernia? • Are There Other Existing Conditions? (diabetes, scleroderma, scoliosis, cerebral palsy, cystic fibrosis, Down syndrome, Sjögren's syndrome, back brace for an unstable spine, recent surgery) • Do You Take Medications That May Aggravate GERD? (antacids, asthma medications, calcium channel blockers, birth control pills, NSAIDs, anticonvulsants, antidepressants, sedatives)

Chapter Three

Asthma • Coughing and Hoarseness • Esophagitis • Strictures and Difficulty Swallowing, Painful Swallowing • Bleeding

Foreword

HEARTBURN—THE word itself is at once innocent and worrisome. Gastroesophageal reflux disease (GERD) is very common, but since the pain is located in the chest it can sometimes raise concerns that the heart is at fault.

Even though GERD is so common, it can be serious, as author Elaine Fantle Shimberg can fully attest. Complications are uncommon but can be severe. The loss of her uncle from esophageal cancer prompted her to research and write this book. Her loss is our gain, however, as the result is a concise informational book that is extraordinarily user-friendly. Complicated medical material has been predigested and simplified.

The spectrum of reflux ranges from babies (severe spit-up can be a sign) to the elderly who regurgitate and aspirate. We are lucky to have good treatments, both good drugs and good surgical approaches, and these are well reviewed in this book. The chapter on stress management is especially useful for anyone with GERD.

All you need to know about GERD is provided here.

— CHRISTINA M. SURAWICZ, M.D.
Chief of Gastroenterology,
Harborview Medical Center, Seattle,
Past president of the American
College of Gastroenterology

G ERD IS a chronic disease." Throughout the text the author stresses this critical message and also provides an excellent treatise on understanding and treating this illness.

Even after thirty years of studying GERD and treating patients, I found the material in this text informative. Ms. Shimberg has an excellent grasp of the multiple aspects of this common and chronic disorder, which should be of great value to the millions of individuals in the United States who suffer from GERD. Starting with the Preface, which describes Uncle Marty and his long bout with the symptoms of GERD, eventually leading to the development of cancer of the esophagus, the author paints a very clear and instructive picture of the clinical presentation of GERD. She also is careful to remind readers that heartburn or persisting chest pain is also a symptom that occurs secondary to a heart attack and thus cautions that the symptom should never be taken lightly and should always be discussed with a physician. I particularly commend the author for the outstanding chapters on GERD in infants and children, medications that may aggravate GERD symptoms, Barrett's esophagus, "myths" concerning GERD, GERD and pregnancy, and the many sections on the various treatments and how to approach physicians who treat this disease.

It was a pleasure for me to have the opportunity to review the material in this text. To those of you who suffer any of the various symptoms or complications of GERD, I highly recommend this very informative and practical guide to your chronic condition.

—DONALD O. CASTELL, M.D.
Kimbel Professor and Chairman,
Department of Medicine,
The Graduate Hospital, Philadelphia,
Past president of the American
Gastroenterological Association

MEDICAL WRITERS tend to be pack rats, tearing out newspaper and magazine articles on health care issues of interest and tucking them away for use in some future article or book. After almost thirty years of clipping, my files are overflowing.

Within the last eight years or so, I began to notice a specific trend: numerous articles in both the lay press and professional journals on heartburn and gastroesophageal reflux disease. Then, in 1996, my professional interest in these disorders took a more personal turn. I saw firsthand what so-called simple heartburn could become.

My uncle Marty was a people person. He loved people, both young and old, and they loved him in return. A self-educated man, he had grown up in New York City, traveled with the USO during World War II, and served as manager to Rocky Marciano, the heavyweight boxing champion of the world. Yet he quickly adopted and became an active member of his new community of Ironton, a small town in southern Ohio along the banks of the Ohio River. There he and his wife raised two sons (my cousins) and ran Edelson's Men's Store, a clothing store that was begun by my grandfather.

In addition to his business, he was an organizer of the Lawrence County Boys Club and had served as president of various organizations including the Lawrence County Youth Council, Ironton Lions Club, Ironton American Legion Post 433, and his synagogue. He spent hours conducting Jewish Sabbath services for prisoners at the nearby penitentiary and giving speeches about Judaism to local service clubs.

Marty loved to eat, even though he often paid for his indulgence with painful attacks of heartburn. When the heartburn continued even between meals, he wrote it off to stress. When his heartburn bothered him, he popped antacids to relieve his symptoms.

"I remember going to the local drugstore in the seventies," his younger son, Mickey, said. "I bought him cartons of cigarettes and boxes of Tums and Gelusil." He kept the antacids everywhere, in his office, his car, in his home, and took them constantly. But the heartburn grew more painful.

Marty began sleeping partially sitting up in a recliner chair because he suffered such great discomfort when he was lying flat in bed. He often had a bitter taste in his mouth. In August 1996, he began to have difficulty swallowing solid food.

Sensing that he might have something more serious than just heartburn, Marty went to see his doctor, who referred him to a gastroenterologist. There he received devastating news. He had adenocarcinoma of the esophagus, a type of cancer with a poor prognosis.

The family traveled to a major swallowing center, a medical facility dealing with swallowing and esophageal disease that is staffed by physicians and speech pathologists with specialized training and experience. After discussing the various palliative measures with the gastroenterologist there, Marty and his family decided against surgery. He opted for esophageal dilation. The specialist placed a metal shunt into Marty's esophagus to keep the passage open enough for food to move through. His diet became restricted first to soft foods, then foods pureed into a mushy preparation in the food processor. But Marty began to lose weight. He tried a macrobiotic diet and other supplements; he saw an acupuncturist. There was no obvious alteration of his disease. His frantic family made him liquid protein shakes to keep his weight up, but it was futile. Just nine months after being diagnosed with adenocarcinoma of the esophagus, at age seventy-eight, Marty Weill died of what he had thought was just plain old heartburn.

Although most cases of heartburn and acid gastric reflux do not end up as esophageal cancer, reflux of stomach acid can do serious harm to the delicate tissues of the esophagus, create constant pain, and adversely affect a person's quality of life. And, as with my uncle, in some cases it can cause adenocarcinoma of the esophagus.

The statistics concerning esophageal cancer are shocking. According to the American Cancer Society, esophageal cancer is the eighth most common cancer worldwide and the sixth most common cause of death from cancer. And adenocarcinoma of the esophagus is on the rise, especially among white males age fifty and older.

Although, in most cases, gastroesophageal reflux disease (GERD) does not turn into esophageal cancer, the risk of its doing so are very real, as I learned from my uncle's experience. My original file on heartburn and GERD has grown to fill an entire file drawer. It no longer is just an "interesting" disease for which I collect data.

I wrote this book to help others understand how to reduce the symptoms of heartburn and to learn the dangers of gastroesophageal reflux disease, so this growing menace can be properly treated before it becomes deadly.

The anecdotes appearing in this book from people with the disorder are their actual words. When requested, I have changed their names and occupations. You can tell when it's a pseudonym because, in those cases, I use only a first name. All other names are real.

Acknowledgments

N**O BOOK** of this magnitude can be written without the input of many people. I was fortunate to have the assistance and guidance of a number of experts—professional health care specialists as well as laypeople who are dealing firsthand with the problems of GERD. All were willing to share their knowledge, advice, and experiences. Many thanks to all of them—both listed and inadvertently omitted—for their invaluable expertise. They include Anne Blomqvist, R.N.; Donald van der Peet, M.D.; William E. Whitehead, Ph.D.; G. Richard Locke III, M.D.; Daniel Van Durme, M.D.; Richard Lockey, M.D.; Beth Anderson; Laura Barmby; La Leche League; Jeffrey H. Peters, M.D.; Wayne Grody, M.D., Ph.D.; Joel Richter, M.D.; and Laurence A. Bradley, Ph.D.

Thanks also to Danny O'Neal and the staff at the University of South Florida Health Sciences Library. Their efforts in teaching me how to locate research over the Internet and to find additional sources of material were outstanding and much appreciated. They were patient and always available.

Morris R. Hanan, M.D., and H. Worth Boyce, Jr., M.D., were most gracious in accepting the task of reading this manuscript for medical accuracy. I thank them both for their time and interest. Any errors still present are my fault, not theirs.

Most of all, I owe a special debt to gastroenterologist H. Worth Boyce, Jr., M.D. He devoted countless hours offering both suggestions and detailed information. He also helped me to reorganize the necessary chapters, which makes this book more accurate and useful. His suggestions, cooperation, and support of this project were invaluable. The success of this book, if any, is due to him. Any errors or omissions are strictly mine.

My gratitude, as always, to my agent, Faith Hamlin, and her colleague, Nancy Stender, both of whom were always available when I had a question and always upbeat when I faltered, fretted, or fussed. I also appreciate the support and input from my wonderful editor at St. Martin's Press, Heather Jackson, and her assistant, Ellen Smith.

As with every book I write, I thank my wonderful husband of thirty-nine years, Hinks Shimberg. As always, he was uncomplaining in having to share our summer vacation in Maine with my stacks of research materials, files, and a laptop computer.

Some people have a foolish way of not minding, or pretending not to mind, what they eat. For my part, I mind my belly very studiously, and very carefully; for I look upon it, that he who does not mind his belly will hardly mind anything else.

— SAMUEL JOHNSON,
in James Boswell's *The Life of Johnson*

Chapter One

Understanding Gastroesophageal Reflux Disease

What Is Gastroesophageal Reflux Disease?

*The more extensive a man's knowledge
of what has been done,
the greater will be his power
of knowing what to do.*

—BENJAMIN DISRAELI

UNLESS YOU'VE been in orbit on a spaceship or lost and drifting at sea for the past few years, chances are good that you've heard of heartburn and gastroesophageal reflux. You can't watch television for more than an hour or so without seeing a commercial for some over-the-counter (OTC) anti-reflux preparation promising that you can eat red peppers with spicy chili, chocolate cake, and black coffee yet still sleep like a baby. Just take their product. The hucksters make heartburn and gastroesophageal reflux (GERD) sound like a piece of cake—chocolate, no doubt. Their thirty- and sixty-second ads often are comedic in tone, making light of this common ailment, with the implication that everybody pops antacids so there's nothing to worry about if you're part of the crowd.

Figures from the American Gastroenterological Association put the "total direct costs of GERD—including all physician services, facility costs, and drug costs—at $9.3 billion in 1998." A research study by Dr. Susan Oliveria and her team discovered that more than $1 billion was spent just on over-the-counter heartburn remedies alone in 1996.

Adding to the confusion of which medicine to take and for what symptom, gastroesophageal reflux is known by a number of names. It is also called acid reflux, reflux, reflux esophagitis, heartburn (which is only one of a number of symptoms of gastroesophageal reflux), esophageal reflux, incorrectly as hiatal hernia, and occasionally by its full name gastroesophageal reflux disease, or by the acronym GERD. (It's known as GORD in Great Britain, New Zealand, and Australia because of the spelling used in those countries, oesophageal.) For the purposes of this book, I use gastroesophageal reflux disease, acid reflux, or GERD.

But what exactly is gastroesophageal reflux disease? It is a potentially serious medical condition in which acid, with or without partially digested food in the stomach, flows backward, up from the stomach, and is regurgitated into the esophagus and sometimes into the mouth. What causes this to happen and what havoc it creates are explained later in this chapter and others.

Heartburn Is Only One Symptom of Gastroesophageal Reflux Disease

Whatever it's called, gastroesophageal reflux can be painful, interfering with the activities of daily living and, in some cases, even turning deadly. Although GERD presents with a variety of symptoms, the one we're all most familiar with is heartburn, a burning, heavy sensation that hits right behind your breastbone and sometimes is accompanied by a bitter taste in your mouth. When heartburn happens, people may head for the nearest hospital emergency department, assuming they're having a heart attack. (Actually, that's a pretty smart step to take. Better safe than sorry. Let the emergency department doctors decide whether you're experiencing heartburn or a heart attack. Sometimes it's even difficult for them to know for sure without conducting some diagnostic tests.)

There's no denying that suffering from frequent heartburn can take all of the fun out of dining. You may have experienced symptoms just as you finish the last of Grandma's Thanksgiving pumpkin pie and pushed away from the dining table or when you're out for pizza. But heartburn also can happen when you bend down to tie your running shoes or when you take a catnap after dinner. It makes you swallow hard and reach for an antacid. According to a study by the United States Surgical Corporation, half the respondents said heartburn had interfered with their work, while 34 percent claimed their heartburn "gets in the way of sex." Heartburn is what some experts call "the Rodney Dangerfield of Medicine," because it gets no respect.

But you're hardly alone. Heartburn affects more than 100 million Americans. The American College of Gastroenterology, a national association representing 6,500 gastroenterologists, reports that more than 60 million Americans suffer from heartburn at least once a month, with more than 10 percent experiencing heartburn daily.

However, heartburn is only one expression of a more extensive and sometimes serious condition called gastroesophageal reflux disease. Statistics from the United States Department of Health and Human Services indicate that more than 7 million Americans suffer from it.

Gastroesophageal reflux affects people of every socioeconomic, ethnic, and religious group (although it seems to be less common among African Americans). GERD knows no age barriers, afflicting infants and the elderly alike, although the greatest incidence (more than 50 percent) is among men and women between the ages of forty-five and sixty-four. Those most likely to have severe cases of GERD are white males over the age of fifty. According to Philip O. Katz, M.D., vice chairman of medicine and chief of gastroenterology at The Graduate Hospital in Philadelphia, "The prevalence of gastroesophageal reflux disease (GERD) has been compared to an iceberg, the bulk of it made up of people who suffer from GERD but never see a health care provider."

No one, it seems, is immune from developing gastroesophageal reflux disease. In 1996 President Bill Clinton learned that his frequent bouts of hoarseness and laryngitis were actually symptoms of GERD.

What Are Other Symptoms of GERD?

While heartburn is the most familiar symptom of GERD, sometimes gastroesophageal reflux creates other problems as well, not only for men and women, but for children and infants too. Sufferers can develop a myriad of medical problems:

- eroded dental enamel caused by the acid reflux
- voice problems such as hoarseness or laryngitis
- difficulty in swallowing (known as dysphagia)
- a repeated feeling of the need to clear the throat
- chronic coughing
- shortness of breath
- postnasal drip
- esophageal bleeding

- ulceration or stricture (narrowing) of the esophagus

- pneumonitis (inflammation of the lungs)

- chest pain

- asthma

- Barrett's esophagus (a precancerous condition)

- esophageal cancer

According to H. Worth Boyce, Jr., M.D., professor of medicine at the University of South Florida College of Medicine and director of the Center for Swallowing Disorders, "Some laryngologists have suggested that acid reflux may play a role as a co-factor with tobacco in the etiology of squamous cell carcinoma of the larynx."

Symptoms in infants and children are somewhat different, such as recurrent vomiting, respiratory problems, and failure to thrive. You can read about these and other symptoms in more detail in Chapter 2.

Asthma also can be both a trigger and a complication of GERD. According to an article in the *Journal of the American Medical Association,* "Epidemiologic evidence suggests that 15 million Americans suffer from asthma, 34% of asthmatic patients have GERD, and up to 40% have peptic esophagitis."[1] An article report in the *Harvard Health Letter Special Report* puts the figure even higher, declaring that 50 percent of people with asthma have GERD.

Untreated, gastroesophageal reflux may create serious complications such as esophagitis, an inflammation of the delicate lining of the esophagus that can lead to bleeding; a narrowing of the esophagus that makes it difficult to swallow; as well as Barrett's esophagus, a premalignant change in the lining of the esophagus that can lead to cancer. Yet, curiously, many individuals, even those with severe cases of Barrett's esophagus, have few symptoms of GERD and actually may be unaware that they have the disease.

Knowledge Is Power

"Knowledge itself is power," claimed Francis Bacon, an English philosopher and author four hundred years ago. And that's the purpose of this book: to help you learn all you can about gastroesophageal reflux disease so you can make educated choices, take the necessary steps to protect yourself and members of your family, and know where to go for quality medical care.

How the Digestive System Works

Things sweet to taste prove in digestion sour.

—SHAKESPEARE, *Richard II*

THE VAST majority of us tend to take our digestive system for granted—that is, we ignore it as long as everything works smoothly (as it usually does). Yet most people have little idea as to the actual workings of the digestive system other than a vague sense of "something in—something out." Even the parts making up the whole of the digestive system remain a mystery to many, as though we were absent on the day that subject was discussed in health class.

While I have no intention of making this a book about the digestive system—fascinating and complex as it is—I think it's important to have this information so we can become aware of what is happening to us when our digestive system malfunctions. This knowledge also aids communication with our health care professional, not only because we can more accurately describe our symptoms to our physician, but also because we can better understand what he or she is telling us in return. It gives us confidence when we have the proper vocabulary and have a basic knowledge of our body's workings.

What Is the Digestive Tract?

The human digestive system is a thirty- to forty-foot-long tube, a spectacular food-processing plant that runs from mouth to anus. Our digestive tract, which is also known as the alimentary canal or colloquially as the gut, incorporates the mouth, pharynx, esophagus (or gullet), stomach, small intestine, large intestine (or colon), rectum, and anus. Each entity performs a different function, with all working together for the successful process of taking food and drink we have ingested, mixing it first with saliva and then other substances to begin the chemical action needed to break the food mass or bolus into tiny particles. It is churned to further break up the particles so the nutrients can be absorbed into the bloodstream, and eight to ten hours later, the waste material the body can't use is unceremoniously dumped. (Although I briefly describe the entire digestive process from beginning to end, readers with gastroesophageal reflux disease will be primarily interested in what happens in the areas from the mouth to the stomach.)

In the Beginning

Our digestive system actually moves into action even before we eat something. Just the aroma of bread baking, the scent of a succulent roast, or the sight or thought of beautifully prepared food can involuntarily get our mouth watering. That happens because our salivary glands have begun to secrete saliva to help moisten our food and to initiate the chemical action needed for the digestive process. As we chew our food (slowly, please), the food mixes with saliva. We swallow, with our tongue forcing the food mass (bolus) to the back of the throat or pharynx, a short, muscular tube.

A rhythmic action of the pharynx muscles carries the bolus down into the second section of the digestive tract, much like the action of a boa constrictor swallowing its prey. This

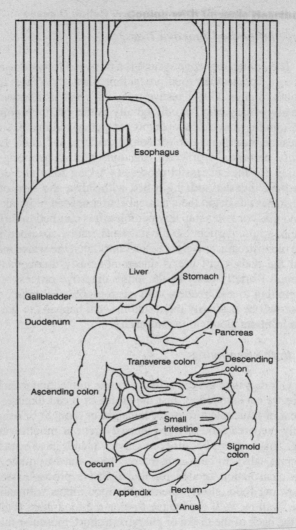

Esophagus

Liver

Stomach

Gallbladder

Duodenum

Pancreas

Transverse colon

Descending colon

Ascending colon

Small intestine

Sigmoid colon

Cecum

Appendix

Rectum

Anus

The Digestive System

Source: National Digestive Diseases Information Clearinghouse, National Institutes of Health.

muscular section is known as the esophagus (from the Greek, meaning "to carry food"). The length of the esophagus varies somewhat among individuals, but usually is about a ten-inch-long tube in an adult. The normal width of the esophagus in an adult is about three-quarters of an inch at the narrowest point. (This dimension is important to remember when someone begins to have difficulty swallowing.) The esophagus lies parallel to and behind the trachea or windpipe. When you choke and say food has gone down "the wrong way," it means that a particle of this food mass has accidentally slipped into the windpipe or trachea on its way to the esophagus.

Food continues to be squeezed down the esophagus and into the stomach by strong rhythmic muscle motions that relax and contract in waves, known as peristalsis or peristaltic movement. When the food mixture gets to the lower esophageal sphincter (LES) or valve between the bottom end of the esophagus and the top of the stomach, the LES opens to permit the flow of the bolus to enter into the stomach. Then, under normal conditions, the LES valve quickly shuts tightly.

The stomach is a J-shaped sac that is the widest part of the alimentary canal. Normally, the stomach can hold about a quart (or a liter) although it can be (and often is) stretched to hold far more. It only takes about eight to ten seconds for this partially digested food mass to reach the stomach, where it is mixed with digestive juice that contains, among other substances, hydrochloric acid (a corrosive substance also found in your car's battery, albeit in lesser proportions).

Normally, the LES closes tightly immediately after the bolus has passed into the stomach. This prevents the food mass from flowing backward into the lower end of the esophagus and up into the throat. When this closing fails to occur, the acid food mixture refluxes, that is, it moves back into the esophagus, burning those delicate tissues, often causing pain and creating a bitter taste in the mouth and throat. We call this discomfort heartburn, the best-known symptom of gastroesophageal reflux.

The Stomach and Beyond

When the LES works properly, the bolus stays in the stomach where it belongs. There the food mass is pummeled by layers of powerful muscles and is tossed like a bundle of soggy clothes in the dryer. But unlike the dryer's action, in the stomach these food particles are further broken down by a combination of the rough tumbling and the addition of gastric juices containing hydrochloric acid and an enzyme called pepsin. When your stomach's upset and you say that you feel as though your stomach is churning, you're absolutely right.

After two to three hours, depending on what you have eaten (fats are digested more slowly than starchy foods), the bolus is mashed, partially digested, and turned into a liquid mush called chyme. Continual peristaltic motion moves this mixture along in squirts through the thick muscular pyloric sphincter at the bottom of the stomach at the rate of two to three teaspoons per minute and into the narrow seventeen- to twenty-foot-long small intestine, which is composed of three parts: the duodenum, the jejunum, and the ileum. It usually takes about four hours for all the food to completely make the journey from the stomach into the small intestine. Additional digestive juices pour into the small intestine from the pancreas, liver, and the walls of the small intestine itself. It is here in these coiled sections of the small intestine that the majority of the absorption of our food nutrients actually takes place.

From the small intestine the remaining mixture, like sludge in a sewer system, moves into the "drying tank," the approximately six-foot-long large intestine or colon. Here, much (80 to 90 percent) of the water component of this waste product is absorbed back into the body. The remaining material—undigested bits of seeds and food fibers, bacteria, bile, and water—moves on into the six-inch rectum, through the one- to two-inch-long anal canal, and out the anus. It is called feces, fecal matter, or just a plain bowel movement.

That's what happens when all is well and your digestive system is working as it should. But many mishaps can occur along the way if one or more of these components fail to function properly, and they can create a baffling number of medical disorders.

What Causes Gastroesophageal Reflux?

A surfeit of the sweetest things
The deepest loathing to the stomach brings.

—SHAKESPEARE, *A Midsummer Night's Dream*

NOW YOU know what is supposed to happen in the gastrointestinal system when there's total harmony. But, unfortunately, sometimes our bodies don't work exactly as described in the anatomy texts. One area of concern to those with heartburn and GERD is the lower esophageal sphincter, a circular muscle located between the esophagus and the upper part of the stomach that acts as a cut-off valve. Normally, this LES valve automatically tightens after food enters the stomach to prevent the food, liquid, and stomach acid from regurgitating or flowing from the stomach back into the esophagus.

But sometimes, for various reasons, this valve doesn't close tightly, or the muscle relaxes slightly. The pressure from the stomach causes the valve to open a bit, permitting a backwash of acidified stomach contents to flow into the esophagus. Although this happens occasionally to almost everyone, it becomes a medical problem when this motion begins to occur more frequently, such as two or more times a week. Then the disorder is called gastroesophageal reflux disease or GERD. (*Reflux* comes from a Greek word that means "backflow.")

This acid seeping into the esophagus and throat can leave a bitter and sour taste in the mouth. More seriously, it causes a burning sensation behind the breastbone that sometimes radiates to the neck, throat, and arms. As the pain often mimics the symptoms of a heart attack, people (wisely) rush to the emergency department to rule out heart disease. It's estimated that of the 6 million people seen annually in hospital emergency departments, 10 to 20 percent of them are experiencing heartburn or GERD, rather than a heart attack.

But don't avoid going to the emergency department because you assume your pain is caused by heartburn and don't want to be embarrassed by making "a big deal" out of your discomfort. Don't try to self-diagnose the symptoms, not even if you're a doctor yourself.

Dr. Sheldon Blau, my coauthor on the book *How to Get Out of the Hospital Alive,* tried to do just that. He's a board-certified physician of internal medicine and a rheumatologist. Nevertheless, when he awoke with the sense of a tight band constricting his chest, he told himself he was suffering from heartburn and took an antacid. It wasn't until the pain moved down his left arm, settling in his wrist, that his denial melted into reality and he went to the emergency department of the very hospital in which he practiced.

While pain triggered by exercise is more likely to be caused by heart disease than heartburn, symptoms of chest pain radiating from the breastbone and into your neck or arm may be difficult to diagnose even by experts. Err on the side of caution. Seek medical help.

What Are Other Causes of GERD?

There are numerous reasons why stomach acid refluxes into the esophagus, throat, and even the mouth. Although I list them briefly here, I deal with them in far more detail in the next chapter.

- A physical weakness prevents the LES from closing.

- A delay in stomach gastric emptying causes the stomach contents to stay longer in the stomach, building up pressure against the LES. This can be caused by medications as well as by other existing medical conditions.

- Normal aging can be associated with LES muscle tone, although GERD is also found in infants and children.

- Diseases such as scleroderma, multiple sclerosis, lupus, and others can cause dysfunction.

- There can be a reduction in the flow of saliva, which usually neutralizes gastric acid in the esophagus. Traces of acid remain in the esophagus longer, burning the delicate tissue. Lack of saliva can be caused by smoking, certain medications, sleeping, and specific illnesses.

- Lifestyle factors, including overeating and overweight, smoking, caffeine, alcohol, and lying down too soon after meals, all may contribute to the LES relaxation, delay in stomach gastric emptying, and a decreased flow of saliva.

- Medications—prescription, over-the-counter, and even herbal remedies—taken for other existing medical conditions can relax the LES resting tone, affect the flow of saliva, and, in some cases, delay stomach gastric emptying.

- Hiatal hernia, while not actually causing GERD, may increase LES relaxation that in turn allows the acid to reflux. A hiatal hernia also may trap or serve as a reservoir for stomach acid, thereby allowing reflux to occur more easily. This permits acid to remain in the esophagus for longer periods, increasing the damage to those tissues.

As you can see, GERD can be caused by a number of factors, which often makes it difficult for the doctor to pinpoint the primary culprit. You need to take an active part in this discovery process and be honest in answering all questions, especially about your drinking, smoking, and eating habits.

How Is Gastroesophageal Reflux Disease Diagnosed?

A disease known is half cured.

—THOMAS FULLER, M.D.

MANY PEOPLE with GERD are walking around with mild or moderate symptoms and have not seen their physician. They're afraid they may be told (and they will be) to stop smoking, stop eating rich or fatty foods, and cut out alcohol and caffeine. So they continue to take over-the-counter medications that temporarily alleviate their symptoms of heartburn, coughing, hoarseness, and wheezing, although these same drugs may also be masking symptoms of a more serious disease. It's also true that some people who have acid reflux have no discomfort at all and none of the traditional symptoms. It's not until they begin to experience difficulty in swallowing (dysphagia) or suffer from chest pains that mimic symptoms of myocardial infarction or angina that they begin to become concerned and make an appointment with their physician.

The fact that you're reading this book—even if a spouse or adult child has pointedly handed it to you or dropped it on your nightstand—probably means that you're having discomfort or even pain from heartburn and that it's been going on for more than a few weeks. Don't keep putting off seeing your doctor. Although this book can tell you a lot about heartburn and gastroesophageal reflux disease, it can't make a correct diagnosis. So pick up the phone and call your doctor today.

While you wait for the day of the appointment to arrive,

get a notebook and start keeping track of symptoms and dates. Our memory is a funny thing. We may think we have total recall, but then we walk into the doctor's examining room and our grasp of pertinent information gaps like the gown we're wearing.

Give a Careful, Thorough, and Honest Medical History

The first thing your doctor will do when you come in complaining of symptoms of GERD is to take a careful medical history. This history is more important than you may realize because it helps the physician to rule out other possible medical conditions. According to Dr. Daniel Van Durme, associate professor and vice chair of the University of South Florida Department of Family Medicine and director of Physical Diagnosis in the USF College of Medicine, "With GERD, 90 percent of a diagnosis is made on history alone. Tests such as an endoscopy [and pH monitoring] can confirm it for you."

Dr. Van Durme also encourages writing down your symptoms in detail, even if you don't think they're too important, so you won't forget any once you get into the examining room. A chronic cough or hoarseness, pain swallowing, a feeling as though food gets stuck in your throat, or wheezing may suggest GERD or even a more serious disease. It's important to be totally honest too, especially when it comes to describing your smoking, illegal drug, and/or alcohol use. Be sure to include information about over-the-counter medications, including vitamin supplements and herbal remedies.

Record how long you've had each symptom and how severe the symptoms are. Is the heartburn merely an annoyance, or is it disrupting your lifestyle? Are you missing work because of your symptoms? Do you awake coughing occasionally, or does the coughing wake you up every night? Do you feel a slight burning in your throat, or is it severe?

Also mention whether you have family members who also

have gastroesophageal reflux disease, as there now is evidence that there may be a genetic disposition to it. "If you have specific concerns," Dr. Van Derme says, "don't wait, holding your breath, hoping the doctor will mention it. If you're afraid you may have esophageal cancer, ask about it straight out."

Because managed care requires doctors to see more patients and spend less time with each patient, you may feel that you still have questions as the doctor begins to edge toward the door. Dr. Van Derme suggests you say, "I want to talk some more about my condition. Is there anyone in your office who could meet with me?" A good doctor should pause long enough for you to ask your remaining questions, or at least have someone in the office who can advise you.

Examination

The doctor will also do a physical exam to rule out other causes of your discomfort and various symptoms, some of which could also point to conditions such as gallbladder disease, coronary disease, or ulcers. Unfortunately, medicine is not an exact science, and often a doctor has to become a Sherlock Holmes as he or she rules out one piece of evidence or puts considerable weight on another.

When Your Symptoms Are Mild

For mild symptoms of gastroesophageal reflux, doctors usually diagnose through treatment, by initially suggesting dietary and lifestyle changes (discussed in Chapter 5) and urging you to use antacids. If you follow these suggestions and your symptoms go away, the diagnosis of GERD was correct. If you still have symptoms, however, or experience pain, bleeding, difficulty swallowing, hoarseness, chronic coughing, or wheezing, your physician will utilize the results of various tests to ascertain if you have something else. With patients over age fifty who also have a long history of symptoms, most physicians prescribe additional tests and plan more aggressive forms of treatment because of the increased incidence of esophageal adenocarcinoma among that age group.

Tests Given to Determine a Diagnosis of GERD

BARIUM STUDIES

This test, called a barium swallow or esophagram, is usually given if you have trouble swallowing or have pain swallowing. You swallow a liquid barium sulfate mixture (which often has been flavored to make the drink more palatable) and then undergo an X-ray examination of your upper gastrointestinal tract. The barium highlights the esophagus so the physician can identify problems such as hiatal hernia, esophageal lesions, or strictures.

Barium studies are not as effective as other tests in making the diagnosis for GERD.

UPPER GI ENDOSCOPY

This test is an important procedure for people with chronic GERD. You are lightly sedated, usually with Versed and Demerol intravenously, and your gag reflux may be depressed with a local anesthetic spray. The physician then inserts a small flexible tube with a light and tiny video camera (endoscope) at the tip down your throat. If you feel anything, it is only a mild sensation. The procedure takes no more than five to ten minutes.

The endoscope enables the physician to inspect the lining of your esophagus to check for inflammation or injuries such as ulcers, erosion, strictures, or the premalignant condition of Barrett's esophagus. If the findings of the endoscopy are abnormal or questionable, the gastroenterologist will take samples of tissue for a biopsy. Your throat may be slightly sore for a day or so afterward.

GASTRIC EMPTYING STUDY

You are given soft food, such as cooked egg whites, containing a radioactive chemical. As you lie on your back, a Geiger counter or camera focuses on your throat and stomach, taking constant pictures for two hours. The purpose is to make sure the stomach is emptying properly. The risk of this exposure to radiation is minimal and, unlike a CAT scan and/or MRI, you don't have to remain motionless.

AMBULATORY 24 PH MONITORING

This procedure is considered the "gold standard" for measuring esophageal exposure to gastric acid. It's one of the more accurate diagnostic tests for GERD.

A tiny, flexible tube called a probe is gently introduced through your nose. It snakes down your throat and passes into your esophagus. There a sensor measures the presence and potency of gastric acidity for twenty-four hours.

The device is taped to your nose, where it remains for one full day. You should eat normally and go about your usual activities, although Scandinavian researchers found that 65 percent of their test patients curtailed their normal routine (probably due to their feeling self-conscious about the probe being so conspicuously taped in place).

If you feel any sign of reflux, you push a button on a Walkman-like recording box that you wear on your belt or on a strap over your shoulder. The box is hooked up to the tubing and monitors the presence of acid in the esophagus. You push another button if you have heartburn or you cough, and yet another when you start and stop eating. You also are asked to keep a chart of when and what you eat, your activity level, and when you lie down or go to bed, as reflux is often worse when you lie down. Although it may hurt to swallow a little because you do sense the presence of the tube, the probe will help to track the times when reflux occurs.

This test is not infallible, however; certain patients with GERD measure a false negative result (simply not have acid reflux during the period of the study).

BERNSTEIN TEST

In this procedure, drops of saline and a mild acid are alternately introduced into your esophagus through a tube inserted into your nose. The purpose of administering the drops is to determine whether the acid drip reproduces symptoms of GERD (and the saline drip brings comfort). It is used infrequently today, as there are more conclusive tests.

ESOPHAGEAL MANOMETRY/MOTILITY STUDY

This procedure tests nerve and muscle functions during swallowing, showing how food moves through the esophagus. A probe is inserted down your nose and into your throat, the upper stomach, and the esophageal sphincter area. You can swallow normally and will be asked to swallow small amounts of water. The esophageal muscle contractions (peristalsis) as well as the pressure and relaxation of the LES are measured at different levels as the probe is slowly retracted. Patients who have undergone this study report that there is some slight residual soreness in both the nasal passages and throat.

The next chapter deals with who may be susceptible to gastroesophageal reflux disease. You may find yourself listed in more than one category.

Chapter Two

Who Is Susceptible to Gastroesophageal Reflux?

Are You Under Chronic Stress?

Take a music-bath
once or twice a week for a few seasons,
and you will find that it is to the soul
what the water-bath is to the body.

—OLIVER WENDELL HOLMES

EVERYONE EXPERIENCES stress to some degree, and it's not all bad. Indeed, the Canadian endocrinologist and stress expert Dr. Hans Selye said, "Stress is the spice of life. . . . Complete freedom from stress is death."

Yet it is well known that continued, unrelieved stress can adversely affect your health, triggering high blood pressure, heart disease, neck and back pain, asthma attacks, and digestive problems, as well as numerous other medical problems. Studies by the National Institute for Mental Health reveal that 70 to 80 percent of all visits to a physician are stress related. Recently, a relatively new field of medicine, called psychoneuroimmunology, has arisen to investigate the connection between the central nervous system and the immune system.

When you're under stress, your body reverts to its prehistoric caveman mode, dubbed by physiologist Walter B. Cannon as the "fight or flight" response. Many changes take place in your body. Among them, the blood vessels in the digestive system narrow, reducing the blood supply to that area and increasing it in your muscles as your body prepares to flee or to do battle with the saber-toothed tiger or neighboring hostile tribes.

Although the saber-toothed tiger is now found only in museums and historical periodicals, your body still prepares the same way for battle, real or imagined. When that tension isn't released, the state of readiness can have harmful effects on your body. Your stomach begins to produce an overabundance of stomach acid. The result is often heartburn and gastroesophageal reflux.

How Stress Affects Gastroesophageal Reflux Disease

Stress is a major player in many diseases of the digestive system, including irritable bowel syndrome, ulcers, ulcerative colitis, and gastroesophageal reflux disease. While stress usually does not actually *cause* the initial problem in most situations, it can be responsible for triggering additional pain and discomfort.

In some deeper level, I think we have always sensed this. Perhaps that's why we subconsciously use terminology that reflects this effect of emotions on our digestive tract when we say, "I was worried sick," "I can't stomach my new boss," "Your behavior nauseates me," or "I have to go by my gut reaction." It's also why many of us tend to lose our appetite when we're upset.

In a recent study by Susan A. Oliveria, Sc.D., M.P.H., of Memorial Sloan-Kettering Cancer Center in New York and colleagues, stress was reported to be an important trigger of heartburn. "Women were 70 percent more likely than men to report stressful family situations and 55 percent more likely than men to report a hectic day at home as causes of heartburn. . . . In contrast, men were 24 percent more likely than women to report a week of long work hours and 50 percent more likely than women to report business travel as causes of heartburn."[1]

There are many anecdotal reports of specific situations where people's emotions have made their GERD symptoms worse. Although most of the evidence connecting stress to the triggering of he   urn and GERD is empirical or discovered through observation, rather than proved scientifically, most physicians dealing with digestive disorders believe in the mind/body connection.

"It's difficult to conduct a scientific experiment to measure the effects of stress on the stomach," said Dr. H. Worth Boyce, Jr., "because in any experiment involving swallowing, the measurement equipment creates stress in itself. We do know that stress increases acid secretions in the stomach and that stress can slow the emptying of the stomach, which allows the acid to remain there longer and makes it more likely to reflux into the esophagus. We also have improved the symptoms of GERD by lowering stress though hypnosis and other stress-reducing techniques."

Perhaps you've had some of these or other similar experiences that triggered heartburn and other GERD symptoms:

- Your presentation ran late so you missed lunch, then you were stuck in traffic, and now you have to dash to catch your plane, so you stuff the rest of a chocolate bar in your mouth and gulp it down. You won't have time to

call your spouse as you'd promised. The pain from
heartburn travels with you.

- It's midnight and you're still working on a report that's
due at 8 a.m. the next morning. You want it to be perfect, to stand out from everyone else's project. You're
relying on black coffee and cigarettes to keep you
awake as you finish editing what you hope are the final
changes. What you'd like to delete are the burning sensations in your throat and mouth

- You've picked up the kids from baseball practice, still
irritated that the coach kept them so late. Now you have
to swing by the drugstore for a prescription, get the dog
from the groomer, and think about something besides
pizza for dinner. Then you remember you promised
your mother you'd stop by her apartment. You wish you
had something to stop the acid reflux.

While you may think that you work best under pressure—
and, indeed, some people seem to—the damage you do to
your body by chronic, unrelieved stress may be serious and
long-lasting. Although stress in itself doesn't cause gastroesophageal reflux disease, it can worsen the symptoms.

Are Type A Individuals More Prone to
Gastroesophageal Reflux Disease?

In the late 1950s, Drs. Meyer T. Friedman and Ray H.
Rosenman, medical researchers who were studying heart
disease, concluded that a specific personality type was more
prone to suffering a heart attack than other personality
types. In their book, *Type A Behavior and Your Heart,* they
coined this personality type as type A and defined it as "an
action-emotion complex that can be observed in any person
who is *aggressively* involved in a chronic, incessant struggle
to achieve more and more in less and less time, and, if re-

quired to do so, against the opposing efforts of other things or persons."[2]

These people with type A personalities thrive on competition and frequently get irritated with others who don't think or act quickly. They are always in a hurry, trying to cram too much into too little time. They eat, speak, move, and think rapidly and fret that everyone else is too slow. They are filled with an extreme sense of urgency and impatience, and they tend to view life as a competitive event for which "going for the gold" and winning it is usually the only measure of success. They have what Friedman and Rosenman called "the hurry sickness." They also often suffer from gastroesophageal reflux disease, although it probably is due to their lifestyle affecting an already existing condition rather than the lifestyle itself.

"I never thought of myself as a type A personality," said a thirty-year-old computer executive. "Then I realized that I was always thinking of my business and usually go to bed at nine so I can get into the office early. I have no hobbies and find it difficult to relax, unless I'm reading trade journals. It's not just the money that drives me, although I consider it a mark of my success; it's the challenge and the competition I love. I guess I'm addicted to the adrenaline rush that comes with it all. I travel constantly with my job, so I often eat airplane fare or grab fast food when the opportunity presents itself. I've always had trouble with my digestive tract and, yes, now that I think of it, I do have many of the symptoms of GERD."

Why Are Type A Individuals Prone to Gastroesophageal Reflux Disease?

While many type A individuals can work long hours, can eat anything that's put in front of them, and have no digestive problems at all, it's not uncommon for people with that type of personality to complain about gastroesophageal reflux as they munch antacids from the economy-size bottles.

Frustration at being kept waiting, anger over a report that's late or incorrect, worrying about not keeping up with the Joneses, or losing at a so-called friendly game of tennis can create intensive internal tension that affects both swallowing and digestion. So can drinking too much coffee or other caffeine-loaded drinks, smoking, wolfing down fast-food meals, eating heavy meals before bedtime, drinking too much alcohol, or indulging in spicy foods. These individuals discover that this self-inflicted stress may increase the amount of acid in their stomach, triggering or at least exacerbating heartburn and gastroesophageal reflux disease.

Time Management Holds Dangers for the Type A Personality

As a nation we are obsessed with time management. Office supply stores, computer stores, and stationery shops are filled with calendars, personal date books, and minicomputer devices, all of which are supposed to help us get to our appointments on time. The Internet bookstore Amazon.com lists more than 1,000 different time management books all advising readers how to utilize their time in more efficient ways to get more done in less time.

These date holders and reminders of what we have yet to do encourage the polyphasic activities (doing two or more things at once) of the type A individual, such as listening to a presentation while making notes for your own project, working on the computer while talking on the phone, or wolfing down a sandwich while working. The tension created by the failure to be successful in both endeavors increases stomach acid and symptoms of gastroesophageal reflux disease, not to mention triggering other significant physical problems such as high blood pressure and heart disease.

You Don't Have to Be a Type A Personality to Suffer from Chronic Stress

Many studies reveal that individuals other than type A personalities suffer from chronic stress. Occupations such as air traffic control, physician, teaching, nursing, and police work tend to create chronic stress, not only because quick and accurate decisions are required but also because of the frustration of ever-mounting paperwork and bureaucracy. But other occupations, such as secretary, administrative assistant, assembly line work, and construction work, also tend to be stress producers. Many researchers feel that this is due to these individuals having no control over their time or workload.

Stressors Can Be Perceived

The cause of stress doesn't have to be real to create problems. Our personal perceptions of an otherwise neutral event can cause immense stress and trigger symptoms of gastroesophageal reflux among other medical problems. What's more, what one person perceives to be a stressful situation, such as a sporting competition or testing procedure, can be exciting or even fun for another.

We can build walls of imaginary tight deadlines to hurdle. While these self-induced time limits may help most people to accomplish their goals, they can create added tension for those individuals who look at missing a deadline as a personal failure, no matter what the cause. Women especially can easily get caught up with scheduling conflicts for children's car pools and elderly parents' doctors' appointments, putting such high demands on themselves that they are doomed to failure. They too often either skip meals, grab fast food, or nibble off their children's plates and then wonder why they suffer from heartburn and gastroesophageal reflux.

We also can create additional stress by worrying about situations that haven't occurred and are even unlikely to, or whose solutions are completely beyond our ability to correct. Mentally playing "what if . . ." can tie you in knots as your body prepares for events conjured up only in your mind.

A 1993 study by Dr. Joel Richter of the Cleveland Clinic and others determined that while stress doesn't actually increase the amount of acid you reflux, it does increase your perception of it.

Certain People in Your Life May Be Causing You Stress

Although some stress results from the way you react to what's going on in your life, more often it comes from people in your life—your boss or coworkers, relatives, and sometimes even your spouse and kids. According to Dr. Ernest Fruge, a psychologist at Baylor College of Medicine in Houston, you need to identify people and situations that might be causing your stress. If it's a family member, he suggests pinpointing the problem and discussing ways to fix what is wrong. For job-related stress caused by a coworker, it often helps to discuss the problem directly with him or her. If that fails, talk with your supervisor or seek help from your company's human resources department. If you can't identify and remedy the cause of your stress, Dr. Fruge recommends speaking with a trusted friend, family counselor, or physician. The important message here is not to let the stress build up. If you can't work things out with a difficult coworker, you need to try to limit your contact as much as possible.

Can People Change Their Reactions to Stress?

Is it hopeless? Can a stress-prone personality be changed or is it "once stress-prone always stress-prone"? The late comedian Henny Youngman is credited with saying, "Death is nature's way of telling a person to slow down." But you don't have to wait for the ultimate red light to shift gears to a slower and less frenetic mode. Experts now claim that type A individuals and chronic worriers have learned their particular behavior style, and for that reason, it also can be unlearned. You need to be constantly aware of instinctive reactions and create intentional new responses to replace those reactions.

Recognize Your Stressful Behavior

Years ago when I was trying to be all things to all people—good daughter, wife, and mother of five while maintaining a successful freelance career—I saw a wonderful cartoon about a circus family. The mother had six arms—one was sweeping, one was cooking, one was diapering the baby, one was helping with homework, and so on. Two toddlers were tugging at her skirts. The caption read, "Hold your horses. I've only got six hands."

I was amused until I realized that I was trying to do the same thing, handicapped as I was with only two hands. That was the moment I realized that I needed to change my responses to life's events.

Recognition of behavior is the first step in moving away from the stress that can affect your health, triggering heartburn and gastroesophageal reflux symptoms. (Later in this chapter, I'll give you specific ways to reduce existing stress.) Once you recognize the signs that make you feel stressed—impatience, anger, helplessness over events, perfectionism, overscheduling, and some polyphasic behavior (thinking or doing more than one thing at a time—multitasking)—you can begin to substitute less stressful behavior.

You may find that you drink too much coffee or caffeine-loaded soft drinks when you're under stress. Recognizing that these drinks make your gastroesophageal reflux worse, you can begin to substitute water or herbal (not peppermint) tea when you're feeling frantic. When you catch yourself trying to do two or more things at once and your heartburn is acting up, remind yourself to slow down and ask the question originally posed by time management expert Alan Lakein: "What's the best use of my time right now?"

Substitute New Responses to Stress-Creating Stimuli

One of the symptoms I quickly recognized in my own behavior was extreme impatience at having to wait in line, in stalled traffic, on the phone, at the doctor's office, and so on. I would sigh, check and recheck my watch, tap my fingers, and get my blood pressure soaring as though I were in a footrace with time. I could actually feel my stomach tighten as I fumed. A few years ago, I decided to take replacement action.

Some of the events that made me impatient were easy to handle. I became more assertive by hanging up the phone when the other person put me on hold and walking out of doctors' offices when kept waiting longer than thirty minutes without an explanation. I kept postcards in my purse and wrote cards to people while waiting in line.

Handling bottleneck traffic was more difficult. Fortunately, someone gave me an audiotape of Robert Frost reading his poetry. I found it very relaxing to listen to the tape and no longer felt angry or frustrated when my car inched along with the others on the road. I even was content to let others pull in ahead of me. I added more poetry tapes to my car collection and still rarely find myself minding a delay in traffic.

What I hadn't realized was that these substitute actions made me feel as though I was in control of the situation. I could read or write postcards rather than stew about a trainee or confused customer holding up a line. I could leave the doctor's office if I felt I had waited long enough, and I could hang up the phone when I tired of being on hold.

Other substitute actions:

- Listen to a musical tape or an author reading his or her poetry or fiction as you walk, rather than review a tape from a conference you missed. (Yes, it's polyphasic behavior, but even relaxed, unstressed folks listen to music as they walk or run.)

- Read a novel or play a noncompetitive game of checkers or Candyland with your kids at night rather than catch up on paperwork.

- Sit in the park and enjoy the swans, squirrels, or just the fresh air as you eat a sandwich or salad from home, rather than gobble down a fast-food burger as you dash to your next meeting.

- Close your mouth when you find yourself beginning to interrupt another person and allow him or her to finish talking before having your say.

- Put down the pencil or move away from the computer during a phone call and concentrate on the call at hand.

- Stop rerunning mental tapes of your past successes and enjoy the moment. Don't let old memories of your high school winning home run or graduating with honors mar your experiencing success as an adult.

- Play a friendly game of softball where the score doesn't really matter instead of joining your buddy for a competitive game of golf.

- Look in a mirror at your desk to catch your expression and when you find yourself frowning, exchange that scowl for a smile.

- Take a ten-minute break in a hectic day just to close your eyes and slow your breathing. Making every moment count doesn't mean you have to be busy every minute. Some of the most precious moments are spent enjoying just being alive.

- Fire the stern taskmaster in your mind and give yourself permission to be less than perfect.

Become aware of how you feel as you consciously change your behavior. Ask your close friends and family to help you check on your progress. You may soon discover that the knots in your neck have loosened, your heart rate and blood pressure are down, and you suffer fewer symptoms of heartburn or gastroesophageal reflux.

There's no doubt that adrenaline-driven individuals often accomplish a great deal. The trick is to strive for and achieve your dreams while still being kind to your body.

It Isn't Your Fault That You Have Gastroesophageal Reflux Disease

You'll just add to your stress level if you've done what you can to reduce stress in your life and feel as though you've failed because you still suffer from heartburn and gastroesophageal reflux. Stop blaming yourself if you suffer from GERD. It isn't your fault, even if you find yourself dealing with a great deal of stress at this point in your life. Although stress doesn't *cause* GERD, it often can aggravate the symptoms of gastroesophageal reflux disease. While following some of the suggested tips can help you to reduce your stress level, they won't cure the medical condition. For that, you need to consult a qualified physician.

GERD Is Not in Your Head

Just because stress can make your heartburn and GERD feel worse, don't think that this means gastroesophageal reflux disease is all in your head. It isn't. It's in your stomach and esophagus. GERD is a real and chronic physical disorder. Although physicians now acknowledge that there is a direct connection between emotions and one's physical condition, that doesn't mean that you're imagining your symptoms. It means that your emotions can and do affect your body.

One of the best-known documented cases that vividly showed the relationship between emotions and the stomach occurred in 1822 when doctors had the rare opportunity actually to see how the stomach digests food. A French Canadian fur trapper was accidentally shot. The resulting injury left a two-and-a-half-inch hole in his stomach. When it healed, the wound was still open, like a window into the interior of the stomach. For the following eight years, the attending physician, an American army surgeon named William Beaumont, was able to observe firsthand how digestive juices work on food and could monitor changes in the stomach lining and alterations in the amounts of stomach acid produced as the trapper's emotions varied.

Despite this knowledge, however, it was some time before physicians and medical schools accepted the connection between the mind and body, agreeing that stress, even perceived stress, could affect our bodies physically. Fortunately, an increasing number of doctors are beginning to acknowledge the interaction between mind and body. An article in *Time* magazine reported that "more and more medical schools are adding courses on holistic and alternative medicine with titles like 'Caring for the Soul.'"

How to Reduce Stress

As I said, although stress in itself does not cause gastroesophageal reflux disease, unrelieved chronic stress can aggravate the symptoms of GERD and make them more severe. For that reason, it's important for you to learn a number of stress-reducing techniques in order to discover which ones work best for you.

I wish I could give you a list of ten ways to reduce stress and you could begin trying them, checking off one and going on to the next. But because each of us is unique and lives a different lifestyle, it's probably going to be a trial-and-error procedure.

One of my sons loves to work in his yard. He is an executive in the high-tech computer world and travels constantly. For him, working with his lawn and flower gardens is a way of unwinding, relaxing, and enjoying himself. This activity also is especially helpful when his GERD is really bothering him and he needs to relax. He says, "Planting and watching things grow is a good lesson in life. There are no 'quick fixes.' You have to invest time and energy into things you want to develop and give them time to bloom. It certainly has lowered my stress level."

I, on the other hand, have no green thumb at all, which was a disappointment to my parents for whom weeding and watering and Miracle-Gro and mulch were favorite dinner-time topics of conversation. Once, when I moved into a new neighborhood, I was asked to join the local garden club where everyone was expected to present some type of floral arrangement. I can't get sweet potatoes to sprout for me, and even my silk flowers droop. I actually got physically sick at the thought of having to create a floral arrangement for others to see. Obviously, I didn't join the garden club.

Almost thirty years ago, when I first was trying to learn some ways to relax and reduce the effects of stress in my life, a therapist tried to help by getting me to visualize myself relaxing as I floated on a cloud. All this exercise ever produced, however, was extreme anxiety. I finally confessed that I had (at that time) a profound fear of heights, and while he was speaking soothing words, hoping to help me to sense a feeling of weightlessness and relaxation, I was tense with worry about falling off that cloud and plunging to an untimely death. Fortunately, he had other suggestions to help promote relaxation, and they have been helpful ever since. So don't be surprised if what relaxes your spouse or best friend doesn't work for you.

EVOKE THE "RELAXATION RESPONSE"

There are many ways to evoke what Dr. Herbert Benson, associate professor of medicine at Harvard Medical Institute and director of The Mind/Body Medical Institute, calls the "relaxation response." They include visualization, yoga, biofeedback, meditation, tai chi, progressive relaxation, music therapy, massage therapy, and even exercise. I'll explore these and other methods of relaxation, and then you can determine what works best for you to help relieve some of the pain you feel from heartburn and other symptoms of GERD. These techniques will not cure your GERD, but they should help you to feel better. They have been tested and found to be worthwhile.

A panel of twelve experts in behavior, pain, and sleep medicines, nursing, psychology, and neurology at the National Institutes of Health concluded that meditation, hypnosis, relaxation, and biofeedback were valid alternative treatments to be used in combination with conventional treatments. According to the panel, "Available data support the effectiveness of these interventions in relieving chronic pain and in achieving some reduction in insomnia." They admitted that the particular approach could vary according to the individual patient.

Your mind and body are not two separate entities. They are one. Training your mind to relax can help your body follow along as well. In his book *Quantum Healing*, Dr. Deepak Chopra states, "A level of total, deep relaxation is the most important precondition for curing any disorder. The underlying concept is that the body knows how to maintain balance unless thrown off by disease; therefore if one wants to restore the body's own healing ability, everything should be done to bring it back to balance."[3]

GUARD AGAINST CREATING MORE TENSION AS YOU TRY TO RELAX

Many people select a hobby or exercise hoping that the activity will help them to relax, but instead find themselves pursing the undertaking with a grim face and a vengeance. We've all seen people "relaxing" on the golf course, steaming when they miss a putt or trying to break a metal golf club over their leg when the ball hits a tree and bounces into the water. While there's nothing wrong with being a little competitive, make sure that you aren't adding to the stress in your life rather than reducing it. If you feel a lump in your throat, heartburn, or even nausea as you bounce around the tennis court, perhaps you should check more than your serve.

Try something different. You don't have to be "good" to enjoy many of these activities. Many highly competitive people have learned to sit quietly in a boat, lazily watching the waves wash over their fish line, not really caring if they catch anything. Others sit at the piano, trying out chords and playing melodies with one finger on their right hand, just letting the sounds of the music ease their tension.

A neighbor of mine treats himself to a new compact disc of either symphonic music or an opera each week. His wife does needlepoint or cross-stitch to relax. Another neighbor took up gourmet cooking to reduce stress. When they entertain friends, he's the one who prepares the meals and we're all pleased to be invited. Others paint, make bread or jam, do wood carving, collect stamps . . . the list is endless. Whatever you decide, it should be relaxing and give you pleasure. If it isn't easily accessible to you when you need it, like sailing, hiking, or horseback riding, just shut your eyes and visualize yourself doing it.

RELAXATION TAKES PRACTICE

Don't get discouraged if you try one or more of these relaxation techniques and they "don't work." It takes practice before you feel less self-conscious and become more proficient. You wouldn't expect to take up a foreign language and immediately speak it fluently or make beautiful music on the guitar on your way out of the music store. Be patient; be kind to yourself.

VISUALIZATION

Visualization is a stress-reducing technique in which you try to re-create in your mind a physical scene that gives you a sense of peace. You focus on this scene using all your senses.

Begin by closing your eyes. Take a deep breath, hold it, then slowly let it out. Repeat twice more. Then let your mind go to a place that fills you with calm. It may be by a gently flowing river, on top of a mountain, or in your garden. Just be sure it's a place that you find beautiful.

My "safe place" is on top of a hill, where I visualize sitting in an old-fashioned rope swing and gently swinging back and forth. Before me is a harbor filled with large sailing ships. I let myself breathe in the salt air as I imagine these tall ships sailing slowly into the harbor. I think the motion of the swing takes me back to my childhood when there was no sense of urgency and I could swing for hours just watching a butterfly fluttering over a flower or finding pictures in the clouds overhead. This visualized scene fills me with a sense of peace and I use it often for five to ten minutes when I feel a need to unwind.

Don't be discouraged when your mind wanders at first. You need to let those thoughts pass by like the clouds overhead and focus again on your special place. It takes practice, but it's an easy way to slip into relaxation mode when you're feeling stressed. If you can find a picture that resembles your spot or an object that you can touch and let that sense carry you back, use it to help you.

PROGRESSIVE RELAXATION

There's nothing magical about progressive relaxation; it actually is relearning a habit you did quite naturally as a baby—when you let your body go limp whenever and wherever you were tired and fell asleep in the car, on the floor, or on a parent's shoulder. The theory is simple: If you are relaxed, you cannot be tense.

Physiologist Edmund Jacobson is considered to be the father of progressive relaxation. In 1929, he described his theory that prolonged tension could trigger certain illnesses. He felt that once someone became aware of tension in a specific muscle group, that person could learn to dispel the tension by relaxing the muscles involved.

There are two forms of progressive relaxation—active and passive—although both have the same goal of creating deep relaxation and freedom from tension. With active progressive relaxation, you lie down and close your eyes. Then, slowly, tense the muscles in your forehead, and focus on what that feels like. Now relax those muscles and be aware of that sensation. Do the same with your cheek muscles, then lips and mouth, neck, and continue working down your body. The purpose of this is that when you feel your jaw tightening or your fingers tensing you will be able to recall the sensation of relaxation in those muscles and be able to release the tension.

Passive progressive relaxation is basically the same, although you do not actually tense your muscles first. Instead, you concentrate on each muscle group, relaxing them as you work up or down your body. Say to yourself, "My toes are relaxed and warm. So relaxed. They float . . ." Work up your body until you reach your forehead. Then think, "Calm," "Jesus," "love," "peace," or any other one word that makes you feel relaxed. This is a "mind message" or mantra. When you focus on your word, you can't think about what you have yet to do at the office or what you're going to do about Billy who's flunking algebra. Your mind can't hold two ideas at one time. If other thoughts do pop in (and it's perfectly natural for them to do so), just let them float on by and think of your word. As I wrote in another book, "Visualize those problems or extraneous thoughts actually moving away from you as though you were a magnet and had reversed the magnetic field, repelling all stressful thoughts and forming a safe protective barrier around yourself. Float, breathe in and out, and relax."[4]

Experts suggest that you practice progressive relaxation at least once a day for ten to twenty minutes in a quiet place where you won't be disturbed. Repeating it a second time each day is even better, but don't practice it more than that. "The idea is not to withdraw from the world," said one psychologist, "but to be equipped to handle stressful situations by being able to relax and release the tension you feel."

EXERCISE

Exercise is a favorite way for many people to relax. But for those with GERD, certain forms of exercise may be counterproductive. It's well known that running or jogging triggers GERD symptoms more than other forms of exercise. According to a study by Dr. C. Scott Clark and colleagues, "running induced the most reflux" even among individuals who did not have GERD normally. This study further suggested that "aerobic exercise with less bodily agitation (bicycle) produced less reflux and may offer an alternate form of exercise for patients with reflux."[5]

There are many other forms of exercise if you have GERD: bicycling, skating, skiing (both water and snow), badminton, volleyball, and perhaps tennis unless it triggers symptoms. Walking is less stressful on joints than running, can be done anywhere, needs no special clothing other than comfortable shoes, seems to trigger fewer GERD symptoms than running, and is a drug-free way to reduce stress. If possible, walk outside to enjoy the beauties of nature.

YOGA AND TAI CHI

Yoga and tai chi are just two of the many ancient forms of relaxation that aid the body by focusing the mind. According to Dr. Andrew Weil, "Some 12 million Americans practice yoga regularly, a number that's *doubled* in the past five years."[6] Both exercises combine specific breathing patterns, posture, and focused attention to help you to maintain both physical and emotional balance. People feel both relaxed and revitalized after yoga and tai chi.

Although numerous videotapes demonstrating yoga and tai chi are available, you should begin by working with an instructor who can teach you how to do the basic moves correctly. Many community centers offer classes in both yoga and tai chi.

MASSAGE

In my opinion, massage therapy is one of the best stress-reducing techniques. In fact, the definition of the word is "the manipulation of the superficial tissues of the body, used for therapeutic purposes and stress reduction." I personally can vouch for the benefits of massage. For the last twelve years, I've enjoyed weekly massages that both relax me and make me feel invigorated. Massage helps relieve the stiffness in my neck and arms and improves my circulation. Massages, however, are not recommended for people who don't like to be touched.

Massage is not a new technique for stress reduction. It was used by both the ancient Greeks and Romans and has been used by Eastern cultures for centuries. Although there are different types of massage, including sports and Swedish, all incorporate some degree of stroking and kneading the body.

Don't expect the massage therapist to be a mind reader, though. Tell him or her what feels good to you. I like a fairly deep tissue massage, while others prefer a lighter, almost feathery touch. Just as you should wait two to three hours after eating before lying down, you should also schedule your massage at least three hours after eating so you don't have problems with reflux. Your lower esophageal sphincter doesn't know if you're lying down in bed or on a massage table.

You can find a qualified massage therapist by checking with a spa, a physical therapist, or a health club. If someone comes to your home, be sure he or she is licensed by your state, if required, and be sure to check references.

BIOFEEDBACK

Biofeedback is a noninvasive therapeutic method that uses electronic monitoring equipment to give information about your brain waves, heart rate, skin temperature, and muscle tension. There is no sensation *from* the equipment to you. It goes the other way; your body sends the information from terminals attached to various parts of your head and body to the machine. The information is revealed back through flashing lights, sounds, or actual visual graphs.

Once you have this information, you can be taught to control your heart rate and muscle tension to reduce your stress level. Biofeedback is used by many psychologists and physicians in dealing with digestive disorders such as irritable bowel syndrome and fecal and urinary incontinence. It is used to a much lesser degree for GERD.

Biofeedback is more expensive than other relaxation techniques, requires a trained person to operate it, and requires you to go to a clinic or physician's office for training.

For free information about biofeedback as well as certified practitioners in your area, send a stamped, self-addressed, business-size envelope to:

The Biofeedback Certification Institute of America
10200 West 44th Avenue, Suite 310

Wheat Ridge, CO 80033
www.bcia.org

MUSIC THERAPY

The English playwright William Congreve wrote in 1697, "Music hath charms to soothe a savage breast, To soften rocks, or bend a knotted oak." Since ancient times, healers have known the therapeutic powers of music to bring people out of their depression, to slow a rapid heartbeat, and to comfort. Present-day researchers have proved the positive effect music can have to control pain. Many surgeons play music in the operating room, well aware not only that their anesthetized patients can still hear but also that these patients usually require less pain medication during recovery.

Music can help reduce your stress level, especially if it stirs up memories of happy times, triggering what Dr. Herbert Benson calls "remembered wellness." Try to select music that has a tempo akin to your heartbeat, approximately seventy to eighty times a minute. Many people use music to help them with progressive relaxation or when they have a massage. I belong to the silent set, finding that music distracts me whether I'm using progressive relaxation, having a massage, or trying to write. On the other hand, just listening to the music does relax me.

But don't just listen to music. Sing, even if you're only a shower singer. According to Dale B. Taylor, Ph.D., director of music-therapy studies at the University of Wisconsin, "Research on brain imaging shows that singing controls the amount of brain activity and slows neural impulses. Singing also helps calm your breathing and heart rate to a normal pace,"[7] which reduces stress hormones. This seems like a good enough reason to add music to your list of relaxation techniques. More than sixty American colleges and universities can't be wrong. They now offer a degree in music therapy as a treatment modality.

MEDITATION AND PRAYER

Meditation and prayer have been used for centuries to help people block out the cares and concerns of the physical world and focus on the spiritual side. Practitioners are able to achieve a state of tranquility and peace, in which breathing, brain wave activity, and heart rate are slowed and blood pressure is reduced. Dr. Herbert Benson says that prayer may lower harmful stress hormones such as adrenaline.

Dr. Bernie S. Siegel writes that spiritual people have higher recovery rates. "They refuse to see themselves as victims," he says. "They also call on God. True peace of mind comes when you have a divine source to help, support, and accompany you, to get you through difficulties and to show you the strength you really have. A relationship with God can help you overcome things that defeat other people."[8]

Although I know of no specific research studies on the effects of prayer on GERD, preliminary results of a study at Duke University Medical Center showed that "people who attend church are both physically healthier and less depressed." It certainly can't hurt to open yourself to the power of prayer, even if you haven't been to church or synagogue since you were dragged there as a child.

LAUGHTER

You may not feel much like laughing when you have the symptoms of GERD, but it is really healthy for you. In his book *Anatomy of an Illness,* Norman Cousins described how he used laughter to help him recover from a serious illness. Numerous other studies show the benefits of laughter, describing how it boosts the immune system and stimulates the brain to release powerful chemical agents called endorphins to help reduce pain.

Laughing makes you breathe deeply, bringing additional oxygen into your lungs. Laughter reduces blood pressure, tension, and pain and improves blood circulation. Laughter lifts the weight of depression. It's hard to be down when you hear laughter.

Charlie Chaplin once said, "Laughter is the tonic, the relief, the surcease for pain." Think about what laughter does for you; think about what it does for comedians. Many of them, like the late George Burns, Jack Benny, Henny Youngman, and Red Skelton, and the present Milton Berle, Bob Hope, and Jerry Lewis enjoyed and are enjoying longevity.

Give yourself time to "wallow in joy," as one woman called it. "I find laughter and happiness," she said, "and wallow in it like a pig back on my daddy's farm."

SEEK HELP

If you've tried a number of the above relaxation techniques and still feel stressed, you may need professional counseling to learn how to deal with the stressors that exist in your day-to-day life. Ask your physician for the name of a qualified therapist in your area.

Are You Pregnant?

*God could not be everywhere
and therefore He created mothers.*

—JEWISH PROVERB

EVEN WHEN it's most welcomed, pregnancy can be stressful. It also makes a woman more susceptible to developing gastroesophageal reflux. I had to look no further than my own family to find an example of this. When I asked my daughter (who was in her seventh month of pregnancy) if she suffered from any heartburn or acid reflux, her answer was a resounding, "Yes! It began immediately."

My daughter's complaint was not unusual. Twenty-five

percent of pregnant women experience daily heartburn and more than 50 percent admit to suffering from heartburn occasionally. That's almost 75 percent of all pregnant women.

What's more, the pattern differs with each pregnancy. One of my nieces, a mother of three, suffered from a burning sensation in her chest with her first two pregnancies. "It began after I ate, regardless of what it was," she said. "I'd take a Tums, and in about fifteen minutes, I'd get relief." In her third pregnancy, however, she experienced no heartburn or gastroesophageal reflux during her first two trimesters. "I thought I was home free," she said with a smile. "Then, in my seventh month, it hit me. Nighttime was the worst. It wasn't any particular food that triggered it, either. After I had the baby, the heartburn stopped."

Obviously, heartburn and acid reflux aren't predictable. One of my daughters-in-law said she had extremely painful heartburn the last trimester with her first child, yet sailed through her entire second pregnancy without a single incidence of heartburn. I had five children and never experienced heartburn. Other women suffer from heartburn and gastroesophageal reflux throughout each day of every pregnancy.

Why Are Pregnant Women More Susceptible to GERD?

There are a number of reasons why expectant women are likely to develop gastroesophageal reflux disease, although it is difficult for doctors to predict which patients are more likely to experience the condition.

HORMONES

When a woman conceives, her hormonal system begins to increase production of a hormone called progesterone. Its function is to prepare the uterus to receive and nurture the fertilized egg.

While progesterone is vital to maintaining the viability of

the fetus, the hormone, along with additional estrogen, also relaxes sphincter muscle tone in the lower esophageal sphincter as well as throughout the entire gastrointestinal tract. When progesterone and estrogen relax the muscles in the digestive tract, they slow down the movement of food so the partially digested mass remains in the stomach longer. This delay offers the opportunity for more nutrients to enter your bloodstream to help nourish your baby. That's the good news.

But the relaxation of the LES also allows stomach acid to seep back up into the esophagus and mouth, causing heartburn and other symptoms of GERD.

PRESSURE

Pressure from the growing uterus as it pushes up against the stomach can also cause GERD. This pressure on the stomach forces the LES to relax just enough to permit regurgitation of the stomach's acidic contents.

TIGHT CLOTHING

Many expectant women, for either economic, fashion, or ego reasons, delay adopting a maternity wardrobe. Their clothing, from the waistbands of their skirts and slacks to their underpants, begins to constrict as their abdomen grows larger. This creates additional pressure on the stomach, enabling the stomach acid to flow backward into the esophagus and mouth.

CONSTIPATION

Constipation, which is defined as the infrequent and difficult passage of stool, also tends to plague many pregnant women. There are many reasons for this. First of all, the hormonal changes that come with pregnancy tend to make digestion slow down. Just as food stays longer in your stomach, waste also lingers longer in the bowel.

In addition, many expectant mothers often drink less water because of nausea experienced in the first (and sometimes second) trimester. Water adds bulk to the stool, which helps it move through the colon. The normal stool is composed of 80 to 90 percent water. Lubrication is due to colon mucus and some stool fat.

Furthermore, the growing fetus puts pressure on the bowel, slowing the peristaltic movement that transports waste material down the bowel and into the rectum. The result is constipation.

When a pregnant woman strains to have a bowel movement, she increases abdominal pressure, which puts added stress on the lower esophageal sphincter. This causes the LES to relax, allowing acid to flow back into the esophagus and mouth.

LYING DOWN IMMEDIATELY AFTER EATING

Because many pregnant women suffer from persistent fatigue, they frequently feel the need to lie down, often immediately after eating. This allows the stomach acid to flow backward from the stomach and into the esophagus and mouth. It's better to rest sitting up in a lounge chair to allow gravity to help keep partially digested food in the stomach where it belongs.

EMOTIONAL STRESS AND FATIGUE

There's no doubt that fatigue is a constant companion to pregnancy, especially if the mother-to-be also holds down a full-time job out of the home, takes care of chronically ill elderly parents, or has other children already in the household. Fatigue coupled with emotional stress—worries about finances, how this baby will fit into the family, how much maternity leave to take, and so on—can also encourage lower esophageal sphincter dysfunction.

What Can Be Done to Reduce Gastroesophageal Reflux?

Fortunately, acid reflux triggered by pregnancy is self-limiting. After the baby's delivery, hormonal levels return to normal, the pressure on the LES is reduced, the stomach empties properly, and the acid backup ceases.

There's no question, however, that gastric reflux disease during pregnancy can be painful, unpleasant, and fatiguing. There's no use suffering unnecessarily. There are steps you can take to reduce GERD while you are pregnant.

- *Wear loose clothing, especially around your stomach.*

Pregnancy is not the time to wear constrictive belts or tight waistbands. If you need to wear hose, get pantyhose especially designed for maternity wear or buy a garter belt that fits loosely on your hips. Tight clothing not only makes you uncomfortable, it also can trigger gastroesophageal reflux disease.

- *Try to relax ten to fifteen minutes before eating.*

Stress at any time can make your gastroesophageal reflux disease more severe. The earlier part of this chapter described in detail ways you can reduce stress in many areas of your life, but an easy way to do so before eating is to take a ten- to fifteen-minute break from whatever you're doing. Focus on slowing your breathing, meditate, or practice visualization. Let your body and mind slow down so when you come to the table, you feel relaxed and able to enjoy your meal.

You may find yourself too tired to grocery shop or to even fix meals. Don't let fatigue add more stress in your life and don't be too proud to accept help. Your husband and extended family members can relieve you of the responsibilities of planning, shopping, and cooking meals, so all you have to do is concentrate on eating them.

Don't grab a bite on the run. You'll pay for it in pain later.

- *Eat frequent small meals, rather than fewer larger ones.*

This may be both easy and beneficial for you, especially if you feel a little queasy during your early pregnancy. Eat often, but not too much at a time. Eat slowly and chew your food well, rather than gulping it down. Avoid drinking beverages with your meals, as the extra volume tends to increase pressure. Take time out to enjoy a healthy snack of fruit, carrots, cheese, raisins, applesauce, a peanut butter sandwich, nuts, crackers, or a yogurt fruit shake around 10 A.M. and another around 3 P.M. Avoid big meals, especially right before going to bed.

- *Eat fruits and vegetables, adding fiber to your diet to prevent constipation.*

Add extra fruit (but not citrus fruit) and vegetables to your diet. They're good for both you and your baby. What's more, they add fiber that helps food move out of your stomach and pass through the digestive tract more quickly. This helps to reduce the severity of your heartburn and lowers the incidence of constipation.

- *Become aware of foods that make your GERD worse.*

Usually, with each pregnancy comes a new list of foods that don't seem too appetizing or that make you feel a little queasy. If you keep a food diary, you may quickly realize that there are certain foods that also make your heartburn worse. Some of them, such as fried foods, spices, and rich desserts (see Chapter 5) are known to weaken the lower esophageal sphincter. Either avoid them during your pregnancy or eat them only in limited amounts.

- *Take a walk after eating.*

Many pregnant women take a leisurely walk after eating. "I don't know if it helped move the food faster," says one, "but the walks certainly eased the acid reflux pain I had been feeling."

Take a stroll, not a jog. Exercise is important when you're pregnant, but avoid strenuous exercise after eating if you want to minimize the effects of gastroesophageal reflux disease.

- *Drink at least eight glasses of water to prevent constipation.*

Be sure to drink at least eight eight-ounce glasses of water daily. Some women remember to do this by carrying a sports bottle of water with them. Others line up eight glasses on the kitchen counter, putting each in the sink or dishwasher after it's been used. Women who work in offices often keep a running total of their water intake on a business calendar or notepad. My sister had a collection of eight miniature pewter pigs. As she finished a glass of water, she moved one of the pigs to the right on her shelf in the kitchen. When all the pigs were on the right, she knew she had "done right" with her fluid intake.

Try different reminders to see what works best for you. Water is important not only to maintain good health but also to reduce constipation and the amount of acid reflux you experience.

- *Try to finish eating dinner at least two to three hours before bedtime.*

Plan your dinner hour early enough so your food has time to digest and there is less in your stomach to reflux when you get into bed. If you're exhausted and feel you must get more sleep, eat earlier or have a light supper. If you have to attend late business meetings where the dinner isn't served until close to your bedtime, plan your heaviest meal at noon.

- *Refrain from bending over whenever possible.*

Squat when you have to pick up things. Wear shoes that don't require tying. When you bend over, you put added pressure on the lower esophageal sphincter.

- *If certain medications seem to trigger GERD, talk to your doctor.*

Certain medications taken for pregnancy itself or for

other existing medical conditions can cause heartburn or other symptoms of GERD. Talk to your doctor about it. Do *not* stop taking the medication without your physician's permission.

If you plan to use birth control pills after the delivery of your baby, be aware that the progesterone in oral contraceptives can trigger the return of GERD in some women, especially those who had severe heartburn during pregnancy.

- *Do not take over-the-counter antacids without your obstetrician's permission.*

Just because a medication is over-the-counter doesn't mean that it necessarily is safe for you to take when you're pregnant. Some antacids, for example, are high in sodium that can dangerously overwork kidneys and cause swelling. Baking soda also is extremely high in sodium and should not be taken while you're pregnant.

Always check with your doctor first before taking something for your heartburn, even if it's an over-the-counter medication or an herbal remedy. Never assume anything is safe to take when you're pregnant. *Check first with your doctor.* Some obstetricians allow their patients to take a calcium carbonate tablet, such as Tums, for relief, while others say no to all antacids.

If, despite all your efforts, you continue to be plagued by symptoms of gastroesophageal reflux disease, look forward to deliverance after delivery. Remember that for most women, GERD disappears (or is minimized) once the baby arrives.

Are You Over Age Fifty?

*A person is always startled when he hears himself
seriously called old for the first time.*

—OLIVER WENDELL HOLMES

THERE'S NO doubt that age creeps up on you, much as
extra weight and inches tend to find their way to your
waist as your years increase. What's more, it always seems
to come as a surprise when you first realize it. I vividly remembered being shocked when, upon congratulating a
group of girls who were about to be confirmed, they replied,
"Thank you, ma'am." I looked around to see just whom they
were talking to.

But the reality of the passage of time really hit home for
me when I recently went to see a new and youngish physician. My bronchitis wouldn't clear up and seemed to be
getting worse each day until I was almost constantly
coughing. The doctor chastised me for waiting so long to
come in. "Don't you know," he railed, "that at your age you
can get dehydrated easily?" I was so shocked to discover I
was at "that age" that I failed to be dismayed about his lack
of tact.

Chances are good that you know an "elderly" person who
complains about heartburn, names a number of foods on the
"can't eat anymore" list, and suffers pain when lying down
after meals. Of course, the definition of what constitutes that
senior section of our population varies widely, often depending, it seems, on the age of the person doing the defining. A
young reporter wrote in the newspaper about an elderly man
being hit by a car. On reading the story I discovered that this
"elderly" man's age was fifty-two.

No matter how old or young you feel and look, as you
pass the half-century mark, you are likely to begin to have
more symptoms of gastroesophageal reflux disease than you
did in your thirties and forties, as GERD does become more

common as people grow older. The severe complications of GERD, especially esophageal strictures, are more common after the age of sixty.

More important, aging on a background of long-term GERD symptoms appears to be a warning sign for increased risk of Barrett's esophagus and esophageal adenocarcinoma.

Why GERD Becomes Worse as We Age

There are numerous reasons why we tend to develop GERD as we get older or, if we already have it, why it worsens.

- *We produce less saliva.*

The salivary glands grow old like the rest of our body and they tend to become less productive as we age. This not only leaves us with a bothersome dry mouth, but it also means that the food we chew has less saliva mixed in with it to moisten it and to help begin the digestive process before the food bolus is swallowed.

- *Peristaltic movement in the esophagus is somewhat decreased.*

Once the bolus is swallowed, older people tend to have less peristaltic movement in the esophagus, so the food tends to move more slowly down the esophagus. When reflux is present, the acid fluid regurgitated into the esophagus doesn't clear quickly and lingers longer against the delicate membrane of the esophagus.

- *There is less muscle tone.*

As this older age group also begins to suffer from reduced muscle tone, once the food passes through the lower esophageal sphincter, the valve often doesn't close tightly. This allows food and acid to reflux into the esophagus. If this reflux occurs at night, the regurgitated material can be aspirated into the lungs, causing pneumonia.

■ *The stomach empties its contents more slowly.*

Because there is a delayed gastric emptying time as we age, our food remains in the stomach longer, where it mixes with acid and is churned longer, making it more likely to reflux.

■ *Medications may aggravate GERD.*

Older people are more likely to take numerous medications—often as many as eight or more a day. These drugs, both prescription and over-the-counter, can intensify existing acid reflux. In addition, the elderly are more likely to suffer from diabetes, Parkinson's disease, heart disease, and respiratory diseases, any one of which may mimic the symptoms of GERD as well as require medications that also aggravate existing gastroesophageal reflux disease.

How Can Adult Children Tell if Older Loved Ones Have GERD?

Adult children of aging parents are often the last to know that their parents have any type of a medical problem. Often their parents don't say anything because they are in denial or they just don't want the expense or bother of taking yet another medication. According to Carol Middlemiss-Weinstock, a gerontological nurse practitioner with Waltham-Deaconness Hospital, "Older individuals often ignore health problems because they desperately want to stay independent for as long as they can, so they minimize their symptoms/problems, and/or prioritize what concerns them most. So they don't always tell you about the GERD symptoms if they have breathing problems or pain that keeps them from walking. And if you think about how many commercials we see about heartburn, people think it's normal."

Middlemiss-Weinstock suggests a number of ways that adult children can tell if their aging loved ones might have GERD. To do so they must have the opportunity to observe their parents or have a friend or neighbor note and relay the information. Here are some obvious signs of GERD.

- belching a great deal after meals

- pain, burning, or general discomfort after meals or when lying down

- sleeping better with more than two pillows (this can also be a symptom of respiratory or heart illness)

- certain foods that "don't agree"

- aversion to foods known to cause symptoms of GERD, such as tomatoes, citrus juices, chocolate, alcohol, caffeine, high fat, or spicy foods

- hoarse or raspy voice (without a history of smoking)

- recurrent bronchial infections

- chronic cough

- chronic sore throat

While these symptoms can be signs of gastroesophageal reflux disease, they also can be symptoms of other potentially serious medical problems. Anyone demonstrating these symptoms should be evaluated by a medical professional.

Are You Overweight?

*More die in the United States
of too much food than of too little.*

—JOHN KENNETH GALBRAITH

IT ISN'T just folks over fifty who are prone to being overweight and therefore more likely to suffer from heartburn and GERD. It's no secret that overweight Americans are on the rise—in percentages as well as in pounds. In fact, according to data from the Third National Health and Nutrition Examination Survey (NHANES III), approximately one-third of all Americans between the ages of twenty and seventy-four are overweight. When you add in the number of people who are not just overweight but are medically considered to be obese, the number becomes a staggering 97 million American adults or 55 percent of our nation's population.

Children Can Be Overweight and Obese Too

It's not just a problem for adults. Unfortunately, children are not exempt from carrying extra pounds, and many of them continue to carry this excess baggage into their adult years. The NHANES III survey reveals that approximately 11 percent or 4.7 million American children between the ages of six and seventeen are overweight. That's more than one in ten children. And their numbers are increasing. Experts suggest that two of the major causes for this added poundage among today's youth are lack of exercise and reliance on fast foods, especially fat-laden hamburgers and french fries. When kids are not lounging in front of the television set or playing computer games, they're being taken through the drive-through window of fast-food eateries by well-meaning parents, the same parents who probably are overweight or obese themselves.

What Harm Is There in Being Overweight?

Most of us know that being overweight or obese is a major risk factor for many disorders including hypertension, type 2 diabetes, arteriosclerosis, osteoarthritis (especially knees and hips), asthma and emphysema, respiratory problems, stroke, and some forms of cancer. Being overweight or obese can cause complications after surgery. Excess weight may also trigger heartburn and other symptoms of GERD in adults and youngsters alike. According to Dr. Donald O. Castell, the key factor may be the type of diet that patients ingest, particularly the fat content. Yet in all the books and magazine articles stressing the need to lose weight, one of the least mentioned problems for overweight people is heartburn and gastroesophageal reflux disease.

How Do You Know if You're Overweight or Even Obese?

Federal guidelines have been set up to identify, evaluate, and suggest treatment for adults who are overweight and obese. (Obesity is defined as being more than 20 percent over "desirable" weight as shown on medical or recent life insurance charts. It is an excess of body fat, whereas overweight is an excess of body weight that includes muscle, bone, and water weight as well as fat.) According to the National Heart, Lung, and Blood Institute, National Institutes of Health, the best way to estimate your total body fat is by finding your body mass index (BMI).

Find your height in the left column of the table on the next page. Look right until you find your weight. The number at the top of that column is your BMI.

According to the federal guidelines, a BMI of 25 to 29.9 is considered overweight. If your BMI is 30 or above, you're considered obese. An exception to this is bodybuilders and similar type athletes who may have a high BMI, but because they have so much muscle and so little fat are still considered to be healthy.

Why Does Being Overweight Trigger Heartburn and GERD?

Extra weight, especially in the abdomen, tends to increase the intra-abdominal pressure around the stomach

Body Mass Index Table

	19	20	21	22	23	24	25	26	27	28	29	30	31	32	33	34	35
Height (inches)	**Body Weight (pounds)**																
58	91	96	100	105	110	115	119	124	129	134	138	143	148	153	158	162	167
59	94	99	104	109	114	119	124	128	133	138	143	148	153	158	163	168	173
60	97	102	107	112	118	123	128	133	138	143	148	153	158	163	168	174	179
61	100	106	111	116	122	127	132	137	143	148	153	158	164	169	174	180	185
62	104	109	115	120	126	131	136	142	147	153	158	164	169	175	180	186	191
63	107	113	118	124	130	135	141	146	152	158	163	169	175	180	186	191	197
64	110	116	122	128	134	140	145	151	157	163	169	174	180	186	192	197	204
65	114	120	126	132	138	144	150	156	162	168	174	180	186	192	198	204	210
66	118	124	130	136	142	148	155	161	167	173	179	186	192	198	204	210	216
67	121	127	134	140	146	153	159	166	172	178	185	191	198	204	211	217	223
68	125	131	138	144	151	158	164	171	177	184	190	197	203	210	216	223	230
69	128	135	142	149	155	162	169	176	182	189	196	203	209	216	223	230	236
70	132	139	146	153	160	167	174	181	188	195	202	209	216	222	229	236	243
71	136	143	150	157	165	172	179	186	193	200	208	215	222	229	236	243	250
72	140	147	154	162	169	177	184	191	199	206	213	221	228	235	242	250	258
73	144	151	159	166	174	182	189	197	204	212	219	227	235	242	250	257	265
74	148	155	163	171	179	186	194	202	210	218	225	233	241	249	256	264	272
75	152	160	168	176	184	192	200	208	216	224	232	240	248	256	264	272	279
76	156	164	172	180	189	197	205	213	221	230	238	246	254	263	271	279	287

To use this table, find the appropriate height in the left-hand column. Move across to a given weight. The number at the top of the column is the BMI at that height and weight. Pounds have been rounded off.

Source: Used by permission of the National Heart, Lung & Blood Institute, National Institutes of Health.

with the extra pressure forcing stomach acid upward through a weakened LES. Once the valve is no longer tight, stomach acid is more likely to flow backward into the esophagus, throat, and mouth.

What Is the Best Way to Lose Weight?

There is no easy way to lose weight. The fad diets that encourage you to eat their food, drink only liquid preparations, or omit a major food group from your diet can be harmful to your health. According to *Current Medical Diagnosis & Treatment,* "There is no special advantage to diets that restrict carbohydrates, advocate large amounts of protein or fats, or recommend ingestion of foods one at a time."[9] Moreover, people who have lost weight on these diets seldom keep the weight off and often gain back even more than they originally lost.

The best way to lose weight is to:

- Check with your doctor before you begin any type of diet and exercise program. Be sure that you really need to lose weight and that it's not your perceived body image.

- Lose weight slowly, no more than two pounds a week.

- Combine "dieting" with at least thirty minutes of exercise three or four times a week.

- Keep a written record of what you eat.

- Drink eight eight-ounce glasses of water each day. You actually retain less water by drinking more. Water helps to lubricate your food as you chew and aids digestion. It also helps to replace fluid lost when you perspire.

- Eat a balanced diet, with special emphasis on fruits and vegetables and limiting foods high in fat or sugar and alcohol. Remember, however, that certain foods may trigger your heartburn and GERD (see Chapter 5).

- Work with an accredited nutritionist, hospital weight-loss program, or nutritionally balanced commercial program such as Weight Watchers that incorporates behavior modification and a support system.

- Ignore over-the-counter medications and herbal preparations that "guarantee" you'll lose weight quickly and easily (often without exercise). If it sounds too good to be true, it is. What's more, it could be harmful to your health.

What if You Are Truly Obese?

If you think you are really obese—and that means a body mass index of 30 or more—what should you do? First, have that diagnosis confirmed by your doctor, not self-determined by reading a magazine article or by looking in a dressing room mirror as you try on a bathing suit. Many people think they are obese when they are really only 5 or 10 percent above the "average" weight on the charts. Remember that "average" does not mean the ideal weight. Your body frame—small, average, or large—may be within that 10 percent range of what's normal. It's when it hits 20 percent or more that you have entered the classification known as obese with all of its potential dangers. If you are medically obese, you really do need to be under a physician's care.

If you are in the obese category, you probably will not be able to lose sufficient weight on your own. Your doctor can help determine if you are eating too much because of depression, lack of exercise, or boredom, or if there is some other medical reason. Then he or she will be able to suggest ways you can begin to safely lose weight. Remember that slow is the way to go when it comes to weight loss. Figure on losing no more than one to two pounds a week.

Whether you are overweight or actually obese, you should find your GERD symptoms easing as you begin to shed some of those extra pounds. Edward Paikoff, a Tampa

Bay periodontist who had suffered from GERD for more than two years, said, "I began working with a personal trainer and lost twenty-two pounds. I haven't had any heartburn or other symptoms of GERD since I lost the weight, and I feel better too. Now I have a double incentive to keep it off." He has kept those extra pounds off for four years.

Infants and Children Can Have GERD

You have to accept whatever comes
and the only important thing is
that you meet it with courage
and with the best you have to give.

—ELEANOR ROOSEVELT

WHEN MOST people think of GERD (if they think of it at all), they tend to think of it as a digestive problem found only in adults. But infants—even newborns—as well as children can and do have gastroesophageal reflux disease. According to Dr. Stuart Abramson, an assistant professor of pediatrics at Baylor College of Medicine and physician at Texas Children's Hospital in Houston, "The most likely cause of cough for children up to eighteen months is gastroesophageal reflux, aortic arch anomalies, or cough variant asthma."

In 1992, pediatric gastroesophageal reflux was classified as a "rare" disorder by the National Organization for Rare Disorders. By 1996, it was considered "one of the most common medical problems in infants. According to Susan Ornstein, a pediatric endocrinologist in Pittsburgh, 5 percent of babies born in the United States have gastroesophageal reflux disease. Vasundhara Tolia, M.D., director of the Division of Gastroenterology, Children's Hospital of Michigan in Detroit, estimates that "the prevalence of GER [gastroesophageal reflux] in normal infants in the first six months of life as reflected by regurgitation range from 18 percent to 50 percent."[10]

How to Know if Your Baby Has GERD

Your infant will quickly let you know if reflux is a problem through a number of signs. He or she may vomit shortly after feeding, regardless if it's breast milk or formula. In fact, gastroesophageal reflux disease is the most common cause of "vomiting" (regurgitation) in infants. But babies can also just spit up—a lot—and have no other symptoms. That makes it difficult to know when to be concerned. How much is too much? When should you worry?

According to Dr. Bruce A. Epstein, a St. Petersburg, Florida, pediatrician with twenty-six years' experience and coeditor of the pediatric Web site www.kidsgrowth.com, "It isn't just spitting up that should give you cause for concern. It's when a baby spits up most of the milk and isn't gaining weight. Infants with gastroesophageal reflux are good eaters," says Epstein. "Many of them are 'guzzlers' and cannot be put off when hungry, finishing their milk very quickly. Other symptoms of reflux might include sudden or inconsolable crying (from the stomach acid), general fussiness, bad breath, and frequent night waking." An Australian study of 102 infants and children age one month to thirty-six months with and without reflux concluded that "Sleep interruption occurs more frequently in infants and children with GORD [GERD] than population norms."[11]

Other experts add to this list of reflux symptoms:

- noisy and difficult breathing
- failure to thrive
- swallowing problems
- arching when feeding as though he or she is trying to get away from the breast or bottle

- frequent burping or hiccuping

- gagging or choking

- poor sleep patterns

- awakens frequently with crying, quickly responds to breast or bottle feeding, then awakens again in one to two hours

- aversion to eating

- aspiration pneumonia

- coughing

- asthma

- sleep apnea

Apnea is a breathing disorder in which the individual temporarily stops breathing for more than ten to twenty seconds. Although adults, especially overweight men, often suffer from apnea, it is extremely frightening when it happens in babies. While over half of all premature babies develop apnea, most of them outgrow it when they reach their term age.

How a Diagnosis Is Made and by Whom

If your baby seems to be spitting up a great deal, especially an hour or so after feeding, or shows any of the other symptoms listed above, see your pediatrician. He or she may want to run some tests to see if reflux is present, or may refer you to a pediatric gastroenterologist.

The doctors may want to schedule an upper GI diagnostic test to check out the baby's upper intestinal tract. This involves giving the baby some chalky liquid called barium to drink. The radiologist follows the progress of this liquid down the digestive tract with fluoroscope and X ray. In children with reflux, the barium can be seen returning up the esophagus. Other tests may include:

- pH probe (see Chapter 1)

- milk scan (scintigraphy), in which a child is fed a radioactive liquid and is scanned to determine how quickly the stomach empties or the liquid is refluxed

- endoscopy, in which a pediatric gastroenterologist looks directly into the esophagus through a tiny flexible scope

Once the diagnosis has been made, the physician will discuss treatment options with you. These may include lifestyle modifications, medication, and occasionally, surgery. Many different medications may be used to treat reflux. They may:

- neutralize stomach acid (such as Mylanta and Maalox)

- reduce acid production in the stomach (such as Tagamet, Pepcid, and Zantac)

- improve intestinal motility (such as Reglan)

- completely block acid production; these medications are called proton pump inhibitors (Prilosec, Prevacid, Nexium, Protonix, and Aciphex)

According to Benjamin D. Gold, M.D., assistant professor of pediatrics, Emory University School of Medicine in Atlanta, "The proton pump inhibitors are a major advance in acid suppression pharmacotherapy and are quite effective in the pediatric age group."

It's important to realize that not all children react the same way to any one drug or to any specific dosage, however. You need to be prepared for some trial-and-error experimentation. Never use over-the-counter medications for your child without your doctor's permission.

How to Feed a Baby with GERD

Your pediatrician can give you some suggestions to make feeding easier for a baby with GERD. One tip is to add a little rice cereal to the baby's formula to make it thicker so it stays down rather than being refluxed into the esophagus. Moms who breast-feed can add breast milk to a little cereal and spoon it into the baby's mouth.

According to La Leche League International, a worldwide breast-feeding support organization, "Breast fed babies with reflux have been shown to have fewer and less severe reflux episodes than their artificially fed counterparts. . . . Human milk is more easily digested than formula and is emptied from the stomach twice as quickly. This is important since any delay in stomach emptying can aggravate reflux. The less time the milk spends in the stomach, the fewer opportunities for it to back up into the esophagus."[12]

Whether breast-fed or bottle-fed, babies with GERD vary in their eating patterns. Some stop eating because they know from experience that they will hurt afterward. Others guzzle their milk down, only to spit most of it back up. Still others sip a bit from time to time because the fluid stops the burning sensation like an antacid. Naturally, this last eating pattern ties the person doing the feeding to an exhausting "on demand" schedule.

The position in which you hold a baby with GERD also is important. Keep the baby as vertical as possible whether you nurse or bottle-feed. That way the milk is more likely to stay in the baby's stomach thanks to the effects of gravity.

Gently burp your baby from time to time throughout a feeding. Take your time. Never rush a feeding, even if you have many other demands on your time, as your baby will sense your tension. Often, just holding and comforting the baby can help to relax him so he's willing to try to eat again.

For those moms wanting to breast-feed their baby with reflux, La Leche League offers a helpful booklet called *Breastfeeding the Baby with Reflux*. You can get it by sending a check or money order for $2.50, made out to La Leche League. Ask for booklet #15. Send a stamped (with two first-class stamps, please), self-addressed, business-size envelope to:

> *La Leche League*
> *PO Box 4079*
> *Schaumburg, IL 60168-4079*

Is There a Genetic Basis for GERD?

Although some researchers are studying a possible genetic basis for GERD, so far none has been found. There does, however, seem to be a family disposition toward GERD. That is, if one or both parents have GERD, there is a strong likelihood that one or more of the offspring will have it too, although this may also be influenced by diet and other environmental factors.

How Long Does GERD Last in Babies?

Most babies outgrow their GERD in six months to a year after birth, although even that reasonably brief period can seem like an eternity to sleep-deprived babies and parents. However, each case is as unique as the baby involved. Some infants continue to have symptoms until their second birthday, and some children continue to have GERD into adolescence and even their teen years.

Having a Baby with GERD Affects the Entire Family

Unfortunately, there's no way that your family will escape being affected if your baby has GERD. But knowing the pitfalls and preparing for them can make life easier for all involved.

THE FATIGUE FACTOR

When your baby wakes often during the night, crying out in pain, you're going to be awakened as well, and the chances are good that you'll be up much of the night, trying to get the baby settled. Somehow it always seems to be worse the night before you have an important meeting or other engagement where you need to be especially alert. There's also an emotional fatigue that sets in as you worry about your infant, wondering if there will be long-term effects from the GERD itself or from the medication the baby's taking to relieve the pain. The emotional fatigue is every bit as real as the lack of sleep.

Don't keep your baby's problem a secret from family and friends. And don't be too proud to accept help. Let friends bring in dinner so you don't have to worry about cooking. Accept the offers from relatives to take the other kids to the zoo or the park so you can look after the baby or even sneak in a nap. Spend time alone with your spouse even if you have to schedule it in your date book. There's no shame in having a baby with GERD, any more than if the baby had any other type of medical condition. When others reach out to help, take their helping hand.

THE TIME CRUNCH

One suggestion concerning feeding an infant with GERD is to give smaller feedings more often. That may work only if the baby doesn't cry for more because the milk has a soothing effect on the irritated esophagus. But feeding takes time. Whether you breast-feed or use formula, it soon seems that all you do is feed this baby, change the diaper, and get ready for another feeding. If the baby spits up often, you also have extra laundry to do and spend additional time wiping off the walls and floor where the spit-up seems to adhere like Super Glue.

Your so-called leisure time tends to evaporate as you struggle to get your baby to stop crying. There's no time for your other kids, friends, or even your spouse, let alone for you. The hands on your clock seem to move in triple time.

You put into effect the suggestion of using gravity to help keep the acid from refluxing by holding the baby almost upright so the milk flows downward. When you do, she's quiet. Holding your breath, you gently put her into the crib, on her back as your pediatrician instructed to prevent SIDS (sudden infant death syndrome). Then the acid spills back into her esophagus, causing her to scream with pain so you have to hold her again. Before long, you feel like screaming too.

GUILT

As parents (especially a mother) of an infant with GERD you feel guilty, even though there's really no reason to. You've done nothing wrong. Nevertheless, there's something wrong with your baby, so in some deep, dark place you feel a responsibility. Maybe it was the glass of champagne you had at New Year's when you were pregnant . . . or the night you made love right before the baby's birth . . . and on you go, searching your mind for some reason that would make sense of why your baby has this painful and exhausting problem. But it *isn't* your fault. Believe that. You're carrying a big enough load trying to cope with a baby with gastroesophageal reflux. You don't need the added burden of guilt. And if anyone tries to lay it on you, turn your back or hang up the phone.

SIBLINGS' RESENTMENT

If you have other children, it's very likely that your older kids feel you spend all your time with the baby and that there's no time left for them. And they may be close to the truth. Soon they begin to resent this noisy intruder who never seems to coo and smile like their friend's new sibling and they wish they had asked for a new puppy instead. You may find your toddler, who was potty trained, suddenly wetting the bed again. If you have school-age children, there may be behavior problems at school.

What can you do to try to unite the family? Communicate with your other children. Too often we parents tend to keep problems to ourselves, not wanting to worry or bother the children with them. But in this case, the siblings feel left out. What's more, in the egocentric way of children, they may feel that they did something wrong and they're being punished by the baby's being sick. So talk to your kids. Explain in age-appropriate terms about gastroesophageal reflux so they'll understand why the baby's in pain and crying. Most likely they'll be more patient and more understanding when they know you're so busy. Perhaps the older ones will be able to help too, so the full responsibility isn't always on your shoulders.

FRUSTRATION LEVEL

There is a tremendous amount of frustration for a parent when you can't seem to make your baby happy. You can understand on an intellectual level about GERD, but emotionally, you feel frustrated and somewhat hurt that you can't make things better. Sometimes you may feel like shaking the baby to make him or her stop crying. Actually, according to experts, the number-one reason a baby is shaken is because of constant crying. *But never shake your baby!* You can do permanent harm. Almost 25 percent of all babies with shaken baby syndrome die.

The National Exchange Club Foundation offers these suggestions to calm yourself when your baby won't stop crying, so you won't do something you'll regret:

- Place the baby in a safe place, like a crib, and leave the room for a few minutes.
- Sit down, close your eyes, and take twenty deep breaths.

- Relax! (See the earlier section in this chapter on ways to relax.)

- Play music.

- Ask a friend or relative to take over for a while.

- Think about how much you love your baby and wouldn't want to do anything to hurt him.

- Don't pick the baby up until you feel calm.

- Make sure the baby is fed and dry.

- Feed the baby slowly and burp her often.

- Gently rock or walk the baby.

- Take the baby for a ride in the stroller or car.

- Check for signs of discomfort such as diaper rash, teething, or fever.

- Call the doctor if you think the baby is sick.

- After immunizations, be sure the baby is comfortable and give recommended medications.

- Put the baby in a windup swing. (Some experts rule out the use of a swing for babies with GERD because it tends to compress the stomach, forcing the acid contents of the stomach into the esophagus.)

- Make sure the baby's clothing is not too tight or that fingers or toes are not bent.

- Give the baby a pacifier.

- Place the baby tummy down across your lap and gently pat or rub the back.

- Offer a noisy toy or rattle.

- Hug and cuddle the baby gently.

- Sing or talk to the baby.

Remember that your baby-sitters, other family members, and extended family can also become frustrated when the baby won't stop crying. Warn them about the dangers of shaking a baby. For more information, contact The National Exchange Club Foundation at 1-800-760-3413. If you have access to the Internet, you can use www.preventabuse.com, or E-mail to info@preventchild-abuse.com. Don't think shaking your child can't happen to you. It can.

LACK OF INTIMACY WITH SPOUSE

The last thing you really feel like is intimacy when you're struggling to calm a baby with GERD. Not that your spouse is probably interested either. You're both too exhausted and frustrated. This is when you look at those childless couples you've been feeling sorry for and a little bit of envy creeps in.

The truth is that you probably need what in my family we call "a little holding time." It needn't be sex, but just the comfort of loving arms wrapped around you, even for just a few seconds. Don't be shy about asking for the comfort hold.

SENSE OF ISOLATION

You may feel like crawling into a dark cave and staying there until this baby with reflux grows up. But this is no time to withdraw from life. Find a baby-sitter who you are sure can handle a crying baby without panicking. (That's probably not your parents or in-laws, even though you'd love them to see firsthand what you've been going through. They may be too close to the situation and take the baby's crying personally.) Get away for even an hour. Go for a walk, play some tennis, or just have lunch with an understanding friend. Give yourself a sense of life outside the GERD arena.

If there's a parent support group such as PAGER in your area, contact them.

PAGER stands for Pediatric/Adolescent Gastroesophageal Reflux Association. They get 10,000 hits a month on their Web site, so you can see that your baby's problem is hardly unique.

PAGER was founded in 1992 by Beth Pulsifer-Anderson, a mom whose daughter had GERD as a newborn and still has it. The organization provides information and support to parents, patients, and physicians. Their board includes parents of children with GERD as well as a number of physicians. The organization's membership roster is international. Although the information on the Web site is free, you can join PAGER for $25 and receive special mailings and a newsletter.

> *PAGER*
> *PO Box 1153*
> *Germantown, MD 20875-1153*
> *Main office: 301-601-9541*
> *West Coast office: 760-747-5001*
> *Web site: http://www.reflux.org/*

There also is a parents' support group in New South Wales called VISA (Vomiting Infants Support Association). Their membership dues are $25 (Australian dollars), which entitles members to approximately sixty pages of information and a bimonthly newsletter. Parents with children who have definitely been diagnosed with GERD may write to receive a complimentary copy of their newsletter. You may write to them at PO Box 4105, East Gosford, N.S.W. 2250.

If there isn't a parents' support group in your community, put a notice in your church or synagogue newsletter or on the community bulletin board, or with your pediatrician's permission, post it in the doctor's waiting room. Chances are you'll find many other parents who also have babies with reflux and thought they were the only ones with the problem.

Hearing others tell of their experiences with a baby with GERD will help you in a number of ways:

- lets you know that you're not alone

- gives you coping strategies that have worked for others

- allows you to laugh at some of the ridiculous situations

- provides new information about research or treatment that you have missed

- creates power in numbers

- promises hope when others describe how their children outgrew reflux or otherwise began to feel better

The Circles of Help

Don't try to go it alone when your infant or child has GERD. The circles of help are intertwined and interdependent. You need to employ each circle to get maximum benefit.

- *Attitude and communication style*

Your attitude and communication style not only helps your family, extended family, and friends, but it also reflects your concern and cooperation with medical staff and when you're dealing with the support group composed of other parents who have similar problems. This doesn't mean that

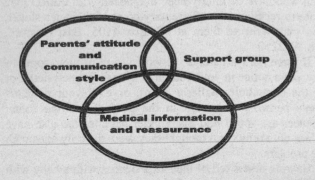

you should affect a cheery disposition when you feel like crying, but rather be honest with your feelings, open to suggestions, and industrious in becoming informed (from reliable sources).

■ *Medical information and reassurance*

Although every parent dealing with GERD wants to absorb as much information as possible about the condition, don't take everything you read or hear as reliable just because you heard it in a chat room on the Internet or from your neighbor at the block party barbecue. Incorrect information circulates just as quickly as valid data.

Check out your expert and his or her credentials. Remember too that in medicine there usually are two (or more) sides to an issue. Medicine is not an exact science, and physicians and researchers often don't agree. That means you may have to sift through the information and, in many cases, go with your gut instinct.

■ *Support group*

Your support group is an important ally when you are dealing with an infant or child with GERD. A support group can be composed of your friends, coworkers, members of your extended family, or just those individuals you have met because their kids also have GERD.

Cut down on interaction with people who give you negative input or who intimate that your child's condition is your fault in some way. First of all, that isn't true and even more important, that kind of talk undermines your self-confidence and impairs your ability to deal with the problems you face. Having a child with a chronic condition is hard enough without having to defend yourself and your actions from those who aren't supportive. Keep your circle of help strong by selecting your supporters wisely.

There's no doubt that having a baby or youngster with GERD isn't easy. Some days it may seem that there is nothing else in your life or mind but reflux. The good news is, however, that the majority of infants outgrow the problem as their body matures and the LES begins to develop more muscle tone so it closes tighter.

For those whose babies continue having GERD into the toddler, preschool, and into adolescence years, you'll soon have enough knowledge to communicate information about it in age-appropriate terms so you can slowly begin to turn the disease over to your child's control.

How GERD Affects a Child as He or She Grows Up

Much of the way a child reacts to a chronic disease depends on how the parents react to it. If the parents are matter-of-fact, the youngster is more likely to take the disease and its treatment in stride, as a part of daily life. As my grandmother used to say when I'd come running to complain about some medical problem, "Everybody's got something. This is what you have." It certainly put things into perspective.

On the other hand, coddling children who have GERD can make them feel different, a state no youngsters want to find themselves in. Encourage normal play activities and exercise. Says Laura Barmby, a parent of a child with GERD, "When my son plays baseball, I see him every so often lift up his head and swallow. I know what's happened. He calls it, 'throwing up in my mouth.' I call it 'adapting to a painful condition.' But he's handling it and I'm proud of him."

For adolescents and teens with GERD, the pain they feel is a constant reminder that they are different from their friends who don't have it. This is accented when it comes to the grazing that young people do today. They know if they join the gang at fast-food restaurants, they're going to pay for it twice, as they also will with carbonated soft drinks, coffee, or an illegal beer. These kids quickly become experts in selecting "safe" foods when they're out with their friends.

If your teenager is on medication, get a plastic pill box at the pharmacy and encourage your child to take charge of keeping track of her pills. Remind her that tight clothes make the reflux worse. Fortunately, the baggy look is in right now.

Encourage your child to tell his friends about the reflux, not for sympathy but rather for understanding. Also urge him to keep up his social life in order to bolster confidence and self-esteem. Isolation just adds emotional pain to the physical pain he may be feeling. Most important, always be willing to give a comforting hug when necessary, but also give your kid a little push to stimulate his independence.

I have a plaque in my kitchen that has faded a little over time, but its message is still clear. It says: "There are only two things we can give our children—roots and wings." It is true with all children, but especially applicable for those with gastroesophageal reflux disease.

Do You Have Asthma?

. . . Find out the cause of this effect:
Or rather say, the cause of this defect;
For this effect defective, comes by cause.

—SHAKESPEARE, *Hamlet*

THE ABOVE quote is very apt because the question of the relationship between asthma and gastroesophageal reflux disease is a circular one, a matter of which comes first, or the question of cause and effect. According to a study by William G. Simpson, M.D., of the Good Shepherd Medical Center in Longview, Texas, "The physiologic effects of airways obstruction and measures used in an attempt to reverse it may worsen GER, or the reflux of gastric contents may worsen or precipitate airways obstruction."

People who are susceptible to GERD—such as those under stress, pregnant women, older people, people who are overweight, and children—are the same individuals who seem to be more susceptible to asthma as well. Asthma is considered to be the most common chronic disease of children and adolescents, and the numbers are increasing, despite newer methods of treatment. Dr. Boris M. Balson and colleagues at Jefferson Medical College in Philadelphia report, "Most children and adolescents with 'difficult-to-control' asthma have abnormal gastroesophageal reflux" as well.[13]

As asthma is also one of the major complications of GERD in addition to being a trigger for gastroesophageal reflux, I am also including information on this disorder in Chapter 3, "Possible Complications of Gastroesophageal Reflux Disease."

People with Asthma Are More Susceptible to GERD

According to Dr. Joel Richter, chairman of the Department of Gastroenterology at the Cleveland Clinic Foundation in Cleveland, "Recent studies have shown that as many as 50 percent to 90 percent of people with asthma also have reflux disease."

Asthma Plus GERD May Prove Dangerous

A study of 260 asthmatics conducted by Dr. Stephen Sontag of Hines Veterans Affairs Hospital in Chicago concluded, "Asthmatics should be especially wary about eating before bedtime . . . it may be a disaster. Nighttime reflux may exacerbate asthma symptoms and vice versa. When acidic material [from the stomach] is refluxed into the back of the throat, it can be inhaled into the lungs. In asthmatics, this can trigger respiratory distress."[14]

You Are an "Expert" on Your Symptoms

Because asthma is often a trigger for GERD, it's important for you to become aware of the various symptoms of acid reflux, although many people—as many as 25 to 30 percent—may have "silent reflux," which is acid reflux without noticeable symptoms. Although approximately 80 percent of asthmatics tested have been found to have an abnormal lower esophageal sphincter, many primary care physicians often don't think of gastroesophageal reflux disease when dealing with their asthmatic patients. For this reason, you need to become an informed and active member of your health care team.

Keep a record of both your asthma and GERD symptoms along with when they appear and what, if known, you think triggered them. Don't trust your memory. Actually get a notebook and write this information down so you can show what you've gathered to your physician. Some hints that you might have GERD:

- nocturnal asthma, which means you wake during the night wheezing, coughing, or even choking

- developing asthma for the first time as an adult

- having more severe asthma after eating or exercising, or when lying down

- having more severe asthma after drinking alcohol

The Medication That Helps Your Asthma May Trigger GERD

Ironically, the very medication that you take to control your symptoms of asthma may be one of the triggers for gastroesophageal reflux disease. Bronchodilator medications (Ventolin and Proventil) and theophylline (Theo-Dur) can make your GERD symptoms worse because the medication relaxes the lower esophageal sphincter. Theophylline also stimulates the stomach to secrete more acid. You'll read more about the effects of these medications as well as others later in this chapter.

Which Is Asthma and Which Is GERD?

Researchers know that there is a chicken-and-egg relationship with asthma and GERD, and physicians often find it difficult to pinpoint just what is triggered by asthma and what by GERD. This interrelationship often creates difficulty for you when you're seeking accurate diagnosis and treatment. That's why you need to help your physician by tracking and reporting your symptoms. This is vital if you or your children suffer from either asthma or GERD. Remember that asthma is a potentially fatal disease if not treated properly, and GERD, left untreated, may become lethal as well.

Does Your Job Require Heavy Lifting, Stooping, or Squatting?

The two kinds of people on earth that I mean
are the people who lift and the people who lean.

—ELLA WHEELER WILCOX

PHYSICIANS AND other health care professionals tend to talk about the deleterious effects of "body positioning" on GERD. What they mean is that specific everyday positions we humans tend to contort our bodies into can compress our stomachs, forcing the acidic contents to back up into the esophagus.

This wisdom is nothing new. In *The Indigestions: Diseases of the Digestive Organs Functionally Treated*, published in 1866, Dr. Thomas King Chambers, honorary physician to England's Prince of Wales, wrote about chest and stomach pain and belching experienced by cobblers. These shoemakers in Victorian times spent up to fourteen hours a day doubled up over their lasts making and repairing shoes. The discomfort was even worse, apparently, among those who "tippled." According to Dr. Chambers, "No greater blessing to the artisan was ever invented than the Upright Shoemaker's Table. . . ."

Ending the Bending

You don't have to be a cobbler to get into positions that compress your stomach. Without thinking, many of us bend over to tie our shoes, pick up an item, or lift a child. Not only is this bad for your back, but it also can intensify reflux and, in some cases, actually force digested material into the throat and mouth. Get in the habit of bending from the knees when you tie your shoes or lift something heavy.

People who garden a great deal also often complain about the frequency of reflux incidents, not realizing that their cramped body position while stooping or squatting can put strain on the LES valve. Suffice it to say, remember the Victorian cobblers. Whenever possible, try to raise your task to eye level so you don't have to compress your stomach.

Avoid Heavy Lifting

Weight lifters, furniture movers, carpet layers, and others whose jobs entail the continual lifting of heavy objects can put added strain on the lower esophageal sphincter as well, forcing stomach acid to regurgitate into the esophagus and throat. I asked a minisampling of three furniture movers if they ever suffered from heartburn during working hours. They looked at me a little strangely. Then they admitted that the problem was considerable, especially when they had an afternoon job right after lunch.

What can you do to prevent reflux? Don't eat heavy meals, drink caffeine products, or ingest other foods that cause you problems just before you have to do work requiring heavy lifting. Loosen your belt and don't wear clothing that constricts your waist or stomach.

Do You Have a Hiatal Hernia?

Anatomy is destiny.

— SIGMUND FREUD

FOR MANY years I overheard the women in my mother's mah jongg group talk about the digestive problems they suffered because of their hiatal hernias. They complained of pain if they ate tomatoes, drank too much coffee, or consumed some other specific type of food. At that time I also considered that hiatal hernia and heartburn were synonymous ailments. But now I've learned that they are not. You can have heartburn and other symptoms of GERD without having a hiatal hernia. It also is possible to have a small hiatal hernia or even a large one that causes no symptoms or discomfort.

What Is a Hiatal Hernia?

If you ever were in a singing or acting class, you may remember being told to breathe from your diaphragm, a large sheet of muscle that separates the stomach from the chest cavity, in order to have better breath control. There actually are exercises taught to develop that type of breathing. I remember my first quarter of college, when I was a theater major, lying on the floor with a book placed over my diaphragm. The instruction was to breathe in and out and watch the movement of the book. (I changed my major before I ever learned to breathe from my diaphragm standing up.)

As you see in the illustration on the next page, there is a small opening in the diaphragm called the diaphragmatic hiatus. Your esophagus passes through this slight cavity and attaches to your stomach just below the diaphragm. A hiatal hernia (also called hiatus hernia) occurs when the upper part

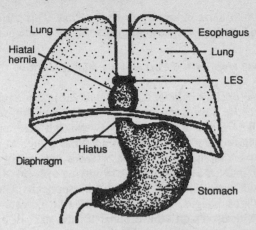

Source: National Institutes of Health

of the stomach slips upward into the chest through this opening. It's estimated that approximately 40 percent of the population has this condition.

Why the Stomach Moves Up into the Chest

Obviously, normally the stomach is supposed to stay where it is—just under the diaphragm. But forceful motions such as coughing, vomiting, or straining at a bowel movement, or a sudden physical exertion such as lifting something heavy, can cause increased pressure in the abdomen. This forces the upper part of the stomach to slip through the opening and slide up into the chest cavity.

Being excessively overweight or pregnant can also cause a hiatal hernia. It is even possible for a hiatal hernia to be present at birth. Fortunately, if this is the case, it often corrects itself without treatment.

Probably the most common contributing factor to the development of a hiatal hernia is the gradual weakening or loosening of the surrounding ligament as we age. This permits increased mobility of the esophagogastric junction region.

What Happens if You Have a Hiatal Hernia

Some doctors believe that a hiatal hernia can trigger reflux because it weakens the lower esophageal sphincter. The hiatal hernia also may allow some stomach acid and partially digested food material in this hernia pouch to collect above the diaphragm. These substances can easily be refluxed into the esophagus, triggering severe GERD, esophagitis (an inflammation of the esophagus), or even Barrett's esophagus. It is estimated that 80 percent of patients with esophagitis have hiatal hernias and all patients with Barrett's esophagus have hiatal hernias.

Is a Hiatal Hernia Age-Related?

Although hiatal hernia is thought by many to be a problem only in middle or old age, this condition actually is found in people of both sexes, and all ages, including adolescents and infants. Babies with a hiatal hernia may regurgitate their food or appear to have trouble swallowing. It is estimated that the majority of otherwise healthy people age fifty and over have a small hiatal hernia but don't seem to be bothered by it.

What Treatment Is Required for a Hiatal Hernia?

Usually, no treatment is required for a hiatal hernia unless severe GERD or esophagitis is present. In that case, medications such as proton pump inhibitors may be prescribed. If, however, the hernia becomes twisted, a rare condition known as strangulation, surgery may be necessary because the constriction can cut off blood supply.

Are There Other Existing Conditions?

Think of the ills from which you are exempt,
and it will aid you to bear patiently those
which now you may suffer.

—RICHARD CECIL

IN ADDITION to the various conditions already mentioned, there are other medical or physical conditions that can make you more susceptible to having gastroesophageal reflux disease. They include, but are not limited to:

- diabetes
- scleroderma
- scoliosis
- cerebral palsy
- cystic fibrosis
- Down syndrome
- Sjögren's syndrome
- back brace for an unstable spine
- recent surgery

Physicians often neglect to tell these patients about the possibility of their developing GERD because they are dealing with other aspects of the disease and aren't focusing on GERD, and with managed care, doctors are limited in the amount of time they can spend with each patient.

Diabetes

One of the little-known complications of diabetes mellitus is gastroesophageal reflux disease. A study conducted by Irene Lluch, M.D., and her team in Spain compared fifty insulin-dependent diabetic patients who showed no symptoms or history of GERD to thirty-six healthy volunteers. The results showed "a higher prevalence (28 percent) of abnormal GERD appeared among asymptomatic diabetic patients than among the general population."[15] This may be related to the slow emptying of the stomach (gastroparesis) associated with diabetic neuropathy, usually in more severe cases.

Scleroderma

Scleroderma, also known as "systemic sclerosis," is a progressive disease causing a hardening and thickening of the skin and also affecting the smooth muscles of the body's organ systems. It is at least three times more prevalent in women than in men.

Scleroderma is another of the medical conditions in which people are also likely to suffer from GERD. That's because the esophagus is composed of a smooth muscle group. According to a Canadian study, as those muscles atrophy and stiffen, "Scleroderma patients suffer a two-fold problem relating to gastro-oesophageal reflux; the lower oesophageal sphincter is an incompetent barrier to an influx of acid from the stomach and they have the inherent clearance difficulties of an aperistaltic oesophagus."[16]

This means that once the stomach acid is regurgitated, it stays in the gullet longer because the peristaltic movement in these patients is lessened. Motility slows. Moreover, the stiffness in the tissues prevent the LES from closing tightly, allowing stomach acid to reflux. Swallowing difficulties also may occur. There also is an increased risk of decreased salivation and dry mouth (xerostomia) with scleroderma, which may aggravate GERD. As the scleroderma patient's muscles begin to atrophy and stiffen, the GERD may become worse. Ironically, some of the medications used to help the other symptoms of scleroderma also reduce the LES tone.

Scoliosis

Scoliosis, curvature of the spine, is a common disorder in childhood that is treated with braces, casts, and often, corrective surgery. Both the braces and casts can put added pressure on the LES, making it easier for reflux to occur.

When scoliosis goes untreated, however, adults may suffer from unequal leg and hip lengths and a painfully twisted spine. This imbalance may put additional strain on the abdomen, which in turn adds pressure to the lower esophageal sphincter, triggering acid reflux. These individuals also are at a higher risk of hiatal hernia.

Cerebral Palsy

Cerebral palsy is a motor function disorder that is most recognizable by the individual's awkward movements and impaired speech patterns. According to researchers, neurologically impaired individuals tend to have many factors predisposing them to severe gastroesophageal reflux. These factors include swallowing problems, hiatal hernia, poor acid clearance, slower esophageal motility, and dysfunction of the lower esophageal sphincter valve.

Cystic Fibrosis

Individuals with cystic fibrosis also are extremely susceptible to GERD because of their chronic coughing that raises their abdominal pressure. That makes them more likely to suffer from hiatal hernia and LES dysfunction as well. According to a review of the literature, Dr. Eric Hassall reported that many families of children with cystic fibrosis (CF) don't report problems of reflux because they consider them to just be a part of the CF. This makes the diagnosis of GERD delayed and, in many cases, may predispose the patient to Barrett's esophagus, a premalignant condition.[17] The delay also may predispose the individual with CF to severe esophagitis and strictures.

Down Syndrome

Individuals with Down syndrome are a very important group to observe for GERD and its complications. They are more prone to problems of GERD because of swallowing problems, hiatal hernia, poor acid clearance, slower esophageal motility, and dysfunction of the lower esophageal sphincter valve.

Sjögren's Syndrome

Sjögren's syndrome, an autoimmune disorder, makes people more susceptible to GERD. One of its many symptoms is dryness of mouth (xerostomia) due to decreased salivation, so acid isn't diluted properly. According to the Sjögren's Syndrome Foundation, up to 73 percent of patients with Sjögren's syndrome have swallowing difficulties. Many of them also have dysfunction in the motility required to get the food bolus into the stomach, so it stays in the esophagus longer. This can cause the esophagus to become inflamed and possibly lead to esophagitis.

Wearing a Back Brace for an Unstable Spine

Individuals who must wear a back brace because of an unstable spine are more susceptible to GERD for the same reason as are people who wear clothes that are too tight. The brace puts added pressure on the LES, which makes it easier for the partially digested food in the stomach to reflux. People with back and torso orthopedic braces and casts also are at added risk for GERD.

Recent Surgery

People who have recently undergone surgery may be more susceptible to symptoms of GERD because of the use of the nasogastric tube used during the surgery. The main problem with the nasogastric tube is that it holds the LES open, allowing seepage or reflux of stomach acid into the esophagus and allowing it to remain longer. This increased dwelling time creates additional esophageal irritation. Refluxed stomach acid can further injure the site and trigger esophagitis. In addition, some patients may have difficulty swallowing after surgery, and the lack of saliva can prevent the acid from being diluted as it normally is.

There are many other disorders that have as a side effect heartburn and other symptoms of GERD. If you suffer from any of the typical or atypical symptoms of GERD, tell your physician. He or she may be so focused on dealing with your primary illness that your problems with acid reflux have gone unrecognized and untreated.

Do You Take Medications That May Aggravate GERD?

O true apothecary!
Thy drugs are quick.

—SHAKESPEARE, *Romeo and Juliet*

MOST OF us take a variety of medicines from time to time, but we tend to compartmentalize them. "This aspirin will make my headache go away." "The theophylline will help prevent or relieve my asthma." "The antihistamine will make my hay fever clear up." Your body, however, doesn't isolate these drugs by individual body system. One medication can and often does adversely affect another existing condition. It also can alter the potency of another drug being taken, either by making it stronger than it should be or weaker. As most people over sixty-five take eight or more medications daily, both prescription and over-the-counter, the chances for drug interactions obviously increase as we get older.

You may not realize that some of the medications you take to control other medical conditions could be partially or greatly responsible for making your symptoms of GERD more severe. Every medication, regardless if it's an over-the-counter nonprescription drug, a prescription medication, or even an herbal "natural" remedy, has certain side effects. Some of these medications trigger symptoms of GERD, while others may cause a dangerous and sometimes even deadly interaction with medication you take to relieve symptoms of gastroesophageal reflux. These drugs also can have serious interactions with other non-GERD-related medications, so always let your doctor know everything you're taking.

Medications for Heartburn

The popular press is greatly responsible for minimizing the potential severity of heartburn and GERD and encouraging the use of various over-the-counter medications to ease discomfort. But they seldom if ever add the warning that OTC antacids are meant to be taken only occasionally, such as a few times every two or three months, and not daily like a vitamin pill over a long period of time. Although instructions written on the bottle or package describe the proper dosage, few of us take the time or have a magnifying glass handy in order to read what's written.

Unfortunately, antacids can mask more serious problems

and give you a false sense of security. The feeling that the heartburn is gone so you're fine can lead to disaster. If taken as directed, for example, antacids containing magnesium can be safe and effective. But many heartburn sufferers begin to think more is better and start popping these over-the-counter medications like candy mints. This excessive use can lead to magnesium poisoning, a condition whose symptoms include clumsiness, weakness, drowsiness, and even coma and paralysis. The most common side effect of antacids containing magnesium hydroxide (milk of magnesia) is chronic, unexplained loose stools or diarrhea.

Older people are especially susceptible to magnesium poisoning from the excessive use of antacids containing magnesium because they tend to process drugs more slowly. They also are usually taking other medications that may interact with the antacids. Others who are more susceptible include those who have had digestive surgery or who are taking medication to slow the digestive system. Such medications include, but aren't limited to, drugs for anxiety, Parkinson's disease, and depression. If in doubt about the safety of taking antacids along with these and other medications, always check with your physician or pharmacist.

Don't think you can dodge the problem by changing to antacids without magnesium and then begin to overuse them instead. While antacids such as Tums are magnesium free, they are high in calcium. If these preparations are used excessively, the overabundant calcium may cause muscle, liver, and kidney problems as well as constipation. Aluminum hydroxide in some antacids (Amphojel) may cause constipation. That's why Maalox and Mylanta are a combination of magnesium and aluminum to counterbalance the diarrhea and constipation side effects.

Check the labels of all over-the-counter medications and take them only as directed. Be sure to ask your pharmacist if there are other medications that may interact badly with the OTC. Even a seemingly harmless medication like Tagamet can cause problems if taken with certain other drugs. Tagamet, a histamine blocker, for instance, should never be taken by people taking Coumadin, a blood thinner. Tagamet is also contraindicated if you are taking Dilantin.

Propulsid (cisapride) was a prokinetic drug that helped move food more rapidly through the digestive system. It was used for nighttime heartburn. Unfortunately, it triggered heart arrhythmias in a number of people, and even fatalities in rare cases when taken along with certain other medications. Propulsid no longer is available in the United States. Another prokinetic drug, Reglan (metoclopramide) is available, although it has side effects in about 25 percent of patients.

Antacids also can affect many prescription drugs by making them either more potent or weakening their effects, so stop thinking of antacids as "harmless." They're medicine, even if you can buy them at the hotel gift shop, the convenience store, or a gas station.

Asthma Medication

Medications containing theophylline relieve asthma (which can be a life-threatening disease) but also can trigger excessive production of stomach acid. Theophylline also tends to relax the lower esophageal sphincter valve, which permits acid to escape from the stomach and flow back into the esophagus. But there can be even more serious side effects. If you also take Tagamet to reduce your stomach acid, the Tagamet can increase the levels of theophylline, sometimes to toxic levels.

According to Dr. Richard Lockey, a Tampa allergist and immunologist, some other medications used for asthma can also cause or increase gastroesophageal reflux. "But don't stop taking the medications," Dr. Lockey warns, "as abruptly stopping any drug is not advisable." Instead, talk to your physician about ways to treat both disorders without seriously impacting the conditions of either one.

Calcium Channel Blockers

Calcium channel blockers such as Cardizem and Procardia can also have a detrimental effect on digestion, even though they may be necessary to treat a heart problem. Again, it's important to continue taking the medication while you discuss the side effects with your physician.

Birth Control Pills

Birth control pills can also aggravate GERD symptoms because the progesterone in them can reduce pressure of the lower esophageal sphincter, allowing the acid-containing stomach contents to reflux into the esophagus and throat. Women who suffered from heartburn and GERD during their pregnancy seem to be most susceptible.

Nonsteroidal Anti-Inflammatory Drugs

Nonsteroidal anti-inflammatory drugs, also known as NSAIDs (Advil, Aleve, or Nuprin), can do much to ease pain, but they also can do a great deal of harm to the digestive system. As with aspirin products, if you take too many of them, they actually can begin to erode the delicate lining of the stomach. When they are not swallowed with a full glass of water, these tablets can stick in the esophagus and ulcerate its lining (a condition known as pill esophagitis).

Nonsteroidal anti-inflammatory drugs are taken daily by thousands of people with arthritis, headaches, menstrual cramps, and aches and pains from trying to be a weekend athlete. It's estimated that "more than 70 million prescriptions and more than 30 billion over-the-counter NSAID tablets [are] sold annually in the United States."[18] Unfortunately, it also is estimated that the "annual number of hospitalizations in the United States for serious gastrointestinal complications [from NSAIDs] is at least 103,000 people."[19] That represents a lot of pain and a great deal of expense.

Medications to Prevent Osteoporosis

If not taken exactly according to directions, Fosamax, a medication used to prevent the crippling effects of osteoporosis, can trigger heartburn and other symptoms of GERD.

Anticonvulsants

Anticonvulsants such as Dilantin, Mesantoin, and Peganone can upset the stomach if not taken according to directions.

Antidepressants

Prilosec may increase blood levels of those also taking Valium and other antidepressants. This means that the antidepressant's action may be prolonged. Your physician may have difficulty regulating your medication because of this interaction.

Sedatives

As sedatives such as Librium, Paxil, and Zoloft tend to slow the stomach's emptying, these drugs may promote acid reflux in susceptible individuals. Ask your physician if there is a substitute medication, but never stop taking any prescribed drug without your doctor's permission.

Do Your Part to Prevent Adverse Drug Interactions

Always tell your physician *every* medication you are taking, regardless if it's prescription, over-the-counter, or even an herbal remedy. Don't think "it's only aspirin," "just a vitamin supplement," "it's natural, just St. John's wort," or "it's only birth control pills."

Unfortunately, many people think that over-the-counter

medications or herbal remedies sold in health food stores are safer than prescription drugs. For this reason, people often use more than the recommended dosages, figuring a little more can't hurt. But it can. As you've read, these and many other medications can be harmful when mixed with other drugs or if you have a specific medical condition. To date, however, there has been little research on the adverse effects of herbal-drug interactions. Many of them undoubtedly exist but remain unknown to you or your physicians.

Nevertheless, it's important for your physician to know everything you're taking, even if it's only eye drops or a vitamin supplement. It's difficult for most of us to remember all the names of medications, especially since most drugs have two names—the brand name and the generic one. The easiest way to prevent problems is to toss all your medications—prescription, OTC, and herbal—into a bag and show them all to your doctor. If the medication about to be prescribed would adversely interact with what you're already taking, your doctor may be able to select another that is equally effective but without the dangerous interactions.

To double-check for safety, whenever you get a new prescription, besides questioning your physician, check with your pharmacist to see if anything you're already taking will interact adversely with the new drug. If you use the same pharmacy for all your prescriptions, your record will be in their computer and they can quickly tell you if there's a possible adverse interaction.

You also can check the *Physician's Desk Reference* in the public library. The lay version is called *The PDR Family Guide to Prescription Drugs*. The *PDR* contains descriptions of all medications with their side effects as well as pictures to show you what each pill looks like. Two other helpful books are *The People's Pharmacy* and *Dangerous Drug Interactions* by Joe Graedon and Teresa Graedon. They contain a great deal of information in an easy-to-read format. You also might want to check *Worst Pills, Best Pills: A Consumer's Guide to Avoiding Drug-Induced Death or*

Illness by Sidney M. Wolfe, Larry D. Sasich, Rose-Ellen Hope, and Public Citizens Health Research Group.

Write to the Council on Family Health and ask for their new free brochure, "How to Prevent Drug Interactions." Send a self-addressed, stamped, business-size envelope to:

> *Council on Family Health*
> *1155 Connecticut Avenue, N.W., Suite 400*
> *Washington, DC 20036*

Unfortunately, the human factor is an important consideration when it comes to your medications. Pharmacies can and do make mistakes when filling your prescriptions. Sometimes it's because the pharmacist can't read your doctor's handwriting (which is why many hospitals now require doctors to type out their prescriptions). Often the name of the drug is too similar to another or, as once happened to me, the pills I was supposed to get sat on the shelf right next to the bottle of the pills I erroneously received. Fortunately, I recognized the mistake before taking the wrong medication. If your medicine looks different from the last time you filled the prescription, go back and question the pharmacist.

In *Dangerous Drug Interactions*, Joe and Teresa Graedon suggest using this safety checklist with your physician and pharmacist:

Dear Doctor/Pharmacist,
To assist me in taking my medicines properly, and to reduce the risk of dangerous drug interactions, please help me answer these questions:

1) What is the name of my medicine?
   brand: _____
   generic: _____
2) What is the dose?
3) What time(s) should I take this medicine?

4) Should I take this medicine:
    __ with food?
    __ at least one hour before or two hours after eating?

5) Are there any special foods I should avoid?

6) Are there any vitamins or supplements I should avoid?

7) Are there any precautions or warnings I should know about?

8) Are there any contraindications that would make this drug inappropriate?

9) Which other medicines should I avoid?

10) Are there any OTC remedies I should avoid?

11) What side effects are common with my medicine?

12) Are there any symptoms that are so serious you would want to know about them immediately?[20]

Team Up with Your Physician

Many of us have coexisting conditions, all of which require medication to cure or comfort us. Therefore, it is vital to work closely with our physicians to be sure that:

- each new prescription doesn't make another condition worse

- one medication doesn't decrease or intensify the effects of another drug

- there isn't a dangerous reaction to whatever else we are taking regardless if it's prescription, over-the-counter, or herbal

While it would be comforting if we could just assume that our doctor remembered what he prescribed the last two visits, plus what other physicians had prescribed, as well as the effects and contraindications of each listed in the most up-to-date PDR, that's a fantasy. There are too many new drugs on the market, too many herbal preparations available, and numerous OTC drugs offered in groceries, in pharmacies, and even on the Web. In addition, today's managed care requires doctors to see many more patients, whisking them away just as we formulate a question or two about a medication.

Making doctor-patient communication even more difficult is that many people find themselves facing a new physician or medical group every time their place of business changes insurance carriers. There is little continuity, and the new physician has a steep learning curve while trying to quickly learn a new patient's medical history, family history, fears, level of learning skills, and cultural taboos, along with the recent complaint, in order to provide quality medical care.

We must join with our physician in cautiously investigating the effects of all the drugs we take, asking pertinent questions and promptly reporting any side effects. Write things down and don't trust them to your memory. Offer information pertaining to your condition. Don't expect your doctor to be a mind reader.

Don't become frustrated if one medicine isn't effective and you have to try another. Remember that each person's body system is unique, and a drug may affect different people differently. Never stop any medication without consulting your physician.

Chapter Three

Possible Complications of Gastroesophageal Reflux Disease

Asthma

The disease and its medicine
are like two factions in a besieged town;
they tear one another to pieces,
but both unite against their common enemy Nature.

— FRANCIS JEFFREY

THERE ARE numerous complications that may be triggered by GERD, some of which are not only very serious but also can be potentially fatal. That's why you need to know what they are and why it's vital to seek medical care early for gastroesophageal reflux so it doesn't progress to a more dangerous state. You sometimes may hear of these complications being called "atypical" or "extra-esophageal."

That means they are outside of what is usually thought of as symptoms of GERD—heartburn, reflux, and pain when swallowing. Nevertheless, they are reported to occur in a major proportion of GERD cases.

One well-known complication of GERD is that of asthma, a potentially serious disease in its own right causing more than five thousand deaths each year. It is estimated that 12 million Americans of all ages suffer from asthma, and that number is growing, both in the United States and in other countries. Depending on which study is cited, researchers conclude that 15 to 85 percent of all asthmatics have GERD either as a major factor or as a coexisting condition.

According to Dr. Joel Richter, chairman of the Department of Gastroenterology, Cleveland Clinic Foundation and the Ohio State University Health Science Center in Cleveland, no one knows for sure exactly how GERD causes asthma. One theory is that the esophagus and the bronchial tubes are positioned so close together in the body that a reaction in one triggers a reaction in the other. "It's pretty well documented that if you put acid in someone's esophagus, the pulmonary tree will tighten to prevent the acid going down the windpipe," said Richter. The other theory is that as acid backs up from the stomach into the esophagus, a little of it seeps into the lungs. "Most studies are pointing toward the idea that these microaspirations of acid into the lungs trigger wheezing, coughing, and swelling, which narrow the airways. This causes the muscles to spasm and creates the asthma attack." This latter explanation may be one of the reasons asthmatics often wake with "nocturnal asthma," because sleeping on your back makes it easier for acid from your stomach to reflux into your esophagus.

The GERD-Asthma Cycle

A major problem with asthma and gastroesophageal reflux disease is that the treatment for asthma often tends to trigger attacks of GERD. It is well known that medications frequently taken for asthma, such as theophylline and some of the inhalers, tend to exacerbate the symptoms of gastro-esophageal reflux by relaxing the lower esophageal sphincter and stimulating gastric acid secretion. According to the American Medical Association, up to 80 percent of asthmatics will have an abnormal lower esophageal sphincter.

Conversely, the material regurgitated into the esophagus when you have GERD can constrict the airways into your lungs, triggering bronchospasms that make you wheeze, cough, and demonstrate the other symptoms of asthma. You need more medicine to help you breathe easier, and that medication triggers more GERD. You begin to travel a vicious circle. Nevertheless, according to a recent study, "Clinical experience has shown that early diagnosis and treatment of GERD often leads to better control of asthma."[1]

Many experts feel that if you have never had asthma before and develop intrinsic asthma (not caused by allergens such as cat hair, dust, mold, and so on) as an adult, there is good reason to believe that you may have GERD.

Children with Asthma and GERD

Children are not immune to either asthma or GERD. Asthma is the leading serious chronic illness of children today, affecting more than 5 million American children under age eighteen. According to a study reported in the *Annals of Allergy, Asthma and Immunology,* "Most children and adolescents with 'difficult-to-control' asthma have abnormal gastroesophageal reflux." The researchers suggest treatment ". . . with recommended doses of H_2 blockers and prokinetic agents [drugs that stimulate gastrointestinal motility to facilitate faster esophageal emptying]," but add that the treatment "has a high failure rate and follow-up studies are essential."[2]

How to Treat Asthma When You Have GERD

First of all, you need to ascertain that you have GERD. According to researchers, approximately 33 to 50 percent of people with asthma have "silent" GERD; they are not aware of having any of the other usual symptoms of gastro-esophageal reflux disease such as heartburn or reflux. Instead, these individuals suffer from the atypical symptoms of asthma, chronic cough, or laryngitis.

If you have asthma, chances are good that you also have GERD. Ask your physician to refer you to a specialist who can make the diagnosis by taking a careful history and performing various diagnostic tests as mentioned in Chapter 1.

Never stop taking your medications for asthma without your doctor's approval. Instead, ask if there are substitute drugs that can help to control your symptoms of asthma without making the GERD worse. Response to medical therapy for GERD in asthmatics may not be detected for three to six months, assuming acid production is adequately suppressed. But clinical experience has shown that once the symptoms of GERD are under control either through medication, lifestyle changes, or surgery (or a combination of these), the symptoms of asthma improve as well.

Coughing and Hoarseness

My hair stood on end
and my voice stuck in my throat.

—VIRGIL, *Aeneid*

FOR MANY years my husband wondered why his voice frequently became hoarse, especially when he was giving after-dinner speeches. He didn't smoke or drink coffee, and drank alcohol only in moderation. Yet he often found himself coughing or clearing his throat and blamed it on one of a number of things—a sinus infection, postnasal drip, cold, or cheering too boisterously for the Tampa Bay Buccaneers. It was both embarrassing and frustrating for him. Knowing that many professional singers and actors also suffered from both of these conditions, my diagnosis was that all he needed was specialized vocal training.

But when I began researching this book, I started to wonder if perhaps his coughing and hoarseness were symptoms of something else, namely, gastroesophageal reflux disease. At my suggestion, he visited a gastroenterologist who, after taking a careful history, performed an endoscopy and discovered that my husband's vocal cords were slightly irritated from refluxed stomach acid. We were flabbergasted, as he had experienced none of the typical symptoms of GERD. The doctor prescribed a proton pump inhibitor called Prilosec, which stops the formation of stomach acid. Since taking the medication twice a day, my husband's coughing and chronic hoarseness have cleared up.

If you have been suffering from a chronic cough or hoarseness (that lasts three weeks or more) and are self-medicating the problem as a cold or sinus problem, you may be misdiagnosing yourself and therefore treating the wrong ailment. You also may be wasting a great deal of time running from doctor to doctor as well as money spent on the wrong OTC or herbal preparations trying to cure yourself. Most people, including some physicians, are not aware that coughing and hoarseness are often the first hints that an individual may have GERD, even if that person has none of the typical symptoms of heartburn or regurgitation. In fact, many people who go to an otolaryngologist (ear, nose, and throat specialist) or a pulmonologist (a specialist dealing with disorders of the lungs) because they have a cough that just won't go away or are suffering from chronic hoarseness are as surprised as we were when the physician diagnoses GERD. Yet according to several researchers, less than half of all patients with GERD-related ear, nose, and throat problems show what we think of as the most typical symptoms of GERD, such as heartburn and regurgitation.

Usually the physician treats such a patient with medication and then, in turn, refers that individual to a gastroenterologist, a specialist who is trained to deal with problems of the stomach and esophagus, to be further tested and treated.

According to a study by Richard S. Irwin, professor and director of the Division of Pulmonary, Allergy, and Critical Care Medicine at the University of Massachusetts Medical School in Worcester, "Postnasal drip syndrome (PNDS), asthma, and gastroesophageal reflux disease (GERD) account for approximately 85 percent of all cases of chronic cough."[3] Other studies "find GERD in as many as 75 percent of patients with chronic hoarseness"[4] and find "20 percent of GERD patients with chronic cough."[5] Regardless of which study is used, it's obvious that GERD should be considered if you suffer from chronic coughing or hoarseness and other factors have been discounted.

How GERD Affects the Voice

The mechanics of the stomach acid working on the vocal cords is very similar to its effects on the airways. When the stomach acid refluxes into the esophagus, it irritates the tissues and triggers the body's cough receptors. The body tries to protect itself by coughing, trying to dislodge the irritant, which it can't. The vocal cords are irritated from both the effects of coughing and the regurgitated acid. Hoarseness results.

The Treatment for GERD-Related Coughing and Hoarseness

Once the physician has ruled out other disorders by taking a careful history, performing a chest X ray and other tests, he or she will prescribe medications along with lifestyle modifications (see Chapter 5) to try to control the coughing and hoarseness. Patience is required on the part of both the physician and the patient, as improvement may take as long as five months. With carefully selected patients, surgery also may be considered as an option (see Chapter 5).

Never neglect a case of chronic coughing or hoarseness. It can lead to more serious disorders.

Esophagitis

> *The pain seemed to be displacing*
> *with its own hairy segments*
> *his heart and lungs;*
> *as its grip swelled in his throat*
> *he felt he was holding his brain*
> *like a morsel on a platter*
> *high out of hungry reach.*

—JOHN UPDIKE, *The Centaur*

ESOPHAGITIS IS inflammation of the lining of the esophagus. It is caused by infection or, more commonly, backflow of gastric juice from the stomach. Esophagitis also can be caused by pills that are swallowed with too little water or while the person is lying down. The pill gets stuck in the esophagus, causing inflammation.

This inflammation or swelling ranges in severity from redness to actual erosions where bleeding takes place and deep ulcers and strictures form. These conditions can cause scarring and a narrowing of the esophagus, which normally is only as wide as a nickel or quarter. Obviously, anything that diminishes that area is going to make eating and swallowing more difficult.

But this continued washing of the esophagus by the gastric juice from the stomach can also develop into an even more serious problem known as Barrett's esophagus, a pre-malignant condition to be discussed later in this chapter. That's why it's extremely important for the physician to determine if you have esophagitis, in order to treat it immediately. The diagnosis can be made with endoscopy (with biopsy, if necessary), which is usually performed by a gastroenterologist. According to Mary P. Bronner, assistant professor in the Department of Pathology at Seattle's University of Washington Medical Center, "The biopsy is not used to rule in esophagitis, but to rule out cancer and Barrett's esophagus."

Individuals with severe esophagitis also may experience some bleeding from the inflamed tissues of the esophagus. Usually, however, any bleeding usually is too slight to be seen, other than under a microscope. It can, however, still cause anemia.

The Treatment for Esophagitis

If you are diagnosed with esophagitis, it is very important that you follow your doctor's instructions, especially those pertaining to lifestyle modifications (discussed further in Chapter 5). This probably means no smoking or drinking alcohol, along with other suggestions. Medication is available for the treatment of esophagitis, and providing you adhere to the physician's advice, your condition should clear up from two to twelve weeks, depending on the degree of severity and the success of the acid suppressors.

In some cases, where scarring has narrowed the esophagus (a stricture), you may have to have that area dilated or stretched in order to permit food and liquids to pass through. You are mildly sedated, then the gastroenterologist slips a dilating tube (dilator) or balloon through an endoscope into the esophagus and gently stretches the area, being careful not to cause undue bleeding in these inflamed tissues.

Don't put off seeing your physician. Conditions such as esophagitis don't heal spontaneously. They only get worse.

Strictures and Difficulty Swallowing, Painful Swallowing

I had most need of blessing, and "Amen"
Stuck in my throat.

—SHAKESPEARE, *Macbeth*

WHILE EVERYONE has an occasional problem swallowing, usually due to eating too fast or being under a great deal of emotional stress, persistent difficulty swallowing (dysphagia) becomes a more serious problem. Dysphagia occurs in many medical disorders, such as Parkinson's, multiple sclerosis, lupus, Lou Gehrig's disease, and stroke. It is also a frequent complaint among those with gastroesophageal reflux disease. The problem sort of sneaks up on you before you realize that difficulty swallowing has become a chronic condition. You may feel as though you have a lump in your throat or that food is sticking in your throat or chest. You may experience a choking sensation when you swallow food.

What Causes Dysphagia?

The primary cause of dysphagia when you have GERD is that the delicate tissues of the esophagus are being constantly bathed with refluxed stomach acid. There also may be motility disorders in which the stomach acid remains longer in the esophagus and is not washed away by the constant rain of saliva. This acid bath can, over time, cause severe scarring as the body tries vainly to heal itself. As scar tissue is thicker than the normal lining of the esophagus, the scarring narrows the inner circumference of the esophagus.

Remember that this area is only about the size of a nickel or a quarter. These places where the space is narrowed are called strictures. They act as barriers to food being swallowed and eventually can actually prevent the bolus and even liquids from making their way down the esophagus and into the stomach. They also can trap pills on their way down to the stomach. It is estimated that nearly 80 percent of esophageal strictures are related to GERD.

How Do You Know if You Have Strictures?

If you've suffered from heartburn and GERD for a long time, you may begin to feel discomfort—first slight, and then becoming more severe—as food passes through the esophagus. You may find yourself chewing longer, washing food down with water or other liquids, and even taking smaller bits of food to help it pass through the esophagus. As mentioned above, you may feel that something is sticking in your throat, suffer chest pain, or become aware of a burning sensation after you've eaten.

Some people change their diets and begin to eat only those foods that slide down easily. As that seems to ease the swallowing problem, they think the condition has been cured and put off seeking medical care. Others with esophageal strictures often tend gradually to reduce their food intake and, as a result, may suffer from weight loss or malnutrition because they are not eating a balanced diet. Some individuals may turn to existing solely on a liquid diet.

If you have silent reflux, however, you may feel nothing unusual until one day food just gets stuck in your esophagus and is vomited up. That means the strictures have greatly blocked your esophagus and you need immediate treatment.

But don't wait for difficulty in swallowing to take place before seeking medical care. Contact your doctor, and before your appointment, make some notes on your symptoms. The Mayo Clinic Health Letter suggests that the following information will help your doctor.

- How would you describe your symptoms? Do you choke or cough on food? Does food stick on its way down? If yes, where does it stick and for how long? Do you ever have food back up?

- How often do you have difficulty swallowing? With every meal? Occasionally?

- Do you have trouble swallowing solids? Liquids?

- Do you have frequent heartburn?

- Do you have pain while swallowing?

- Does food or stomach acid back up into your throat?

- When did your symptoms begin? Are they getting worse?

- Have you lost weight? How much?*

How Strictures Are Treated

Gastroenterologists diagnose strictures by using a barium esophagram in which the barium outlines the size and location of the stricture or strictures. They also use endoscopy to evaluate the situation visually.

Gastroenterologists are able to provide relief for swallowing problems by carefully dilating or stretching the wall of the esophagus to allow food and liquid to pass through. Dilation can be performed on an outpatient basis. You will probably be given what is called "conscious sedation." This is an intravenous medication, usually Versed,

Reprinted with permission from Mayo Clinic Health Letter.

that will make you drowsy, lower your anxiety level, and keep you free from pain. However, you still will be able to respond to the doctor's directions to swallow and so on. The procedure consists of inserting a slender instrument called a bougie or a thin tube with a special balloon attached into the esophagus and gradually gently stretching the inner wall so food and liquid will be able to pass through. It may require a few sessions until the wall is stretched enough.

The physician also will probably prescribe lifestyle modifications as well as a proton pump inhibitor, as studies have shown that aggressive therapy using this acid-suppression medication helps to reduce the need for additional dilations, thus lowering the opportunities for esophageal perforations, infections, bleeding, and other complications. It also offers cost benefits.

Many larger hospitals, especially those connected to medical schools, have special units, often called Swallowing Clinics, that are staffed with experts trained to handle more serious swallowing disorders. Some of the major clinics are listed in the Resources section of this book. Check to see if there is such a facility in your area.

Chronic Swallowing Disorders Are Serious Business

If you suffer from regular symptoms of dysphagia, don't postpone a visit to your physician. The problem can be treated, but earlier is obviously better than waiting until you can't get any food down or you start to vomit it. More important, swallowing disorders may be the sign of a more serious medical condition, including esophageal adenocarcinoma, so check out the problem as soon as you feel discomfort.

Bleeding and Ulcers*

Yet who would have thought
the old man to have had
so much blood in him?

—SHAKESPEARE, *Macbeth*

MANY OF us are familiar with rectal bleeding that comes from hemorrhoids, which are enlarged veins in the anus and rectum that can rupture and produce bright red blood. But bleeding can come from any of the areas of the digestive tract, including the esophagus and stomach.

How Is Bleeding from the Digestive Tract Discovered?

Sometimes bleeding from the digestive tract is obvious. You spit up blood, or you see it in the toilet or on the toilet tissue after having a bowel movement. When there is bleeding in the esophagus, stomach, or duodenum, the stool is usually black or tarry. But you also can have digestive tract bleeding without being aware of it. That's called occult or hidden bleeding. Fortunately, there are ways to discover occult bleeding.

HEMOCCULT II

One of the ways to find occult blood is the Hemoccult II test. Your physician may have given you the packet as part of a routine physical. Although the Hemoccult II is primarily used to check for occult blood that may be caused by colo-

Much of the information in this section was adapted from material from the National Digestive Diseases Information Clearinghouse. It is used with permission.

rectal cancer, it also reveals blood coming from any source in the digestive system.

The Hemoccult II test involves your dabbing a small amount of stool onto squares located on a specially prepared card. You do this for three consecutive days and then mail it back to the doctor or a laboratory. There are specific dietary restrictions for two days before taking the test and during the test, but they aren't too onerous. Your doctor will explain them to you, and they also are written on the packet.

ANEMIA

You may learn from a simple blood test that you are anemic. This means you have a lower than normal hemoglobin count, which is the compound in your blood that disperses oxygen from your lungs into your body's cells and carries the carbon dioxide from the cells back to the lungs. Symptoms of anemia include weakness, fatigue, light-headedness, pallor, and often, headache. Often people go to the doctor because they feel tired all the time or suffer from frequent dizzy spells and only then learn that they're suffering from anemia.

Although many factors cause anemia, loss of blood is one of them. Once your physician learns that you are anemic, he or she will prescribe a number of tests to learn what is causing your anemia in order to treat it.

How Acid Reflux Causes Bleeding in the Digestive Tract

If the bleeding originates in the esophagus, it may be caused by an inflammation at the lower end of the esophagus near the stomach, which is called esophagitis (see page 103). The refluxed stomach acid continually bathes the delicate membranes of the esophagus. Eventually, the acid eats away at the lining. The exposed capillaries begin to bleed.

Bleeding from the stomach can be triggered by alcohol or medications used to treat other conditions, such as aspirin,

aspirin-containing medicines, and various other preparations such as those used for arthritis.

According to the National Digestive Diseases Information Clearinghouse, the most common source of bleeding from the upper digestive tract is ulcers in the duodenum, the upper part of the small intestine. Researchers now believe that these ulcers are caused by excess of stomach acid and infection with *Helicobacter pylori* bacteria.

Although digestive system bleeding is caused by various other diseases, including colorectal cancer, and polyps, those types of bleeding described above are all triggered by too much stomach acid on tissues, which eventually weaken and bleed.

How the Doctor Discovers the Site of the Bleeding

Your physician will take a complete medical history and conduct a physical examination. Symptoms such as changes in bowel habits, stool color (to black and tarry or red), and consistency of stool, as well as pain or tenderness, will tell the doctor which area of the GI tract is affected.

ENDOSCOPY

A common diagnostic technique that allows direct viewing of the bleeding site is endoscopy, which is done through the use of an illuminated, thin, flexible tube that is inserted in the mouth or nose and coaxed down the esophagus and into the stomach. Because the endoscope can detect lesions and confirm the presence or absence of bleeding, doctors often choose this method to diagnose patients with acute bleeding. In many cases, the physician is able to use the endoscope to treat the cause of the bleeding as well.

ANGIOGRAPHY

This technique uses dye to highlight blood vessels. The procedure is most useful in situations when the patient is acutely bleeding: the dye leaks out of the blood vessel and identifies the site of bleeding. In some situations, angiography allows injections into arteries of medicine that may stop the bleeding.

How Bleeding in the Digestive Tract Is Treated

The use of endoscopy has grown and now allows doctors not only to see bleeding sites but also to directly apply therapy. A variety of endoscopic therapies are possible in treating GI tract bleeding.

Active bleeding from the upper GI tract can often be controlled by injecting specific chemicals into a bleeding site with a needle introduced through the endoscope. A physician can also cauterize, or heat treat, a bleeding site and surrounding tissue with a heater probe or electrocoagulation device passed through the endoscope.

Once bleeding is controlled, medicines are often prescribed to prevent recurrence of bleeding. Medical treatment of ulcers to ensure healing and maintenance therapy to prevent ulcer recurrence can also lessen the chance of recurrent bleeding. Studies are now underway to see if elimination of *Helicobacter pylori* prevents the recurrence of ulcer bleeding.

What to Do if You Discover GI Bleeding

Never shrug off the signs of bleeding, assuming it's just hemorrhoids. Bleeding anywhere in the digestive tract is a symptom of a digestive problem. Delay may cause the problem to intensify, sometimes with fatal outcomes. Always see your physician at the first sign of GI bleeding.

Dental Problems

Be true to your teeth,
or your teeth will be
false to you.

—DENTAL SAYING

IT COMES as a surprise to many people that the discovery that their GERD is causing complications occurs during a routine visit to their dentist. Yet, according to an article reported in the *Journal of Oral Rehabilitation,* "It is well known that acid regurgitated from the stomach into the mouth will erode teeth."[6]

The damage, known as dental erosion, can be detected by the naked eye and is different from what we think of as a typical cavity caused by bacteria found in plaque. This type of destruction is prevalent not only in those with GERD but also people suffering from bulimia nervosa, the eating disorder in which individuals force themselves to vomit what they've eaten. The principle is the same: Stomach acid washing into the mouth erodes enamel on the teeth.

In some cases, the dental erosion is so severe that the teeth actually are worn down and shortened, sometimes as much as half their normal height. The erosion can also increase spaces between the teeth. Because the acid eats away at the tooth enamel, the nerve inside becomes more sensitive to hot or cold foods.

Richard Masella, D.M.D., says that "GERD can affect both the appearance and health of teeth. When you have reflux, your teeth are getting a frequent acid bath, and if you've taken a high school chemistry class, you know how potent hydrochloric acid can be. Reflux allows the acid to have both time and exposure on the teeth. The result is the attrition of the enamel." In one study, more than 83 percent of patients with dental erosion referred by dentists for testing were found to have GERD.[7]

As the lower front teeth usually are only slightly affected by the acid, you may not realize the amount of destruction going on it your mouth until it is too late. That's a good reason to have regular dental checkups, especially if you suffer from GERD.

Barrett's Esophagus

In the face of uncertainty,
there is nothing wrong with hope.

— BERNIE SIEGEL, *Love, Medicine and Miracles*

BARRETT'S ESOPHAGUS. It certainly sounds benign enough. The name almost has a lyrical quality to it (reminds us of Elizabeth Barrett Browning, perhaps?). But there's nothing beautiful about Barrett's esophagus. It was named for British surgeon Norman Rupert Barrett, who described the lesion in 1950. Barrett's esophagus (BE) is also known as Barrett's metaplasia and columnar-lined esophagus. Whatever you call it, BE is a nasty disease, a sign of GERD going wild. It is a precancerous condition occurring in approximately 10 to 15 percent of those who have GERD and 40 percent or more of those with acid reflux–related strictures.

What's more, cases of Barrett's esophagus are expanding dramatically. According to Douglas Levine, M.D., with Astra-Xeneca, the incidence of Barrett's esophagus has tripled over the past twenty years. James C. Reynolds, M.D., and colleagues at the Division of Gastroenterology and Hepatology at MCP Hahnemann University in Philadelphia reported, "Patients with Barrett's metaplasia carry an increased risk for the development of esophageal adenocarcinoma that is 30 to 125 times that of an age-matched population. It has been estimated that 700,000 to 1.5 million Americans have Barrett's metaplasia."[8]

What Is Barrett's Esophagus?

As you remember from Chapter 1, the stomach is protected from being burned by its own acid because of its special lining called columnar epithelium. *Columnar* refers to the type of cells, and *epithelium* refers to the cells that make up the lining and covering of the body's organs.

The mucous membrane that lines the esophagus, on the other hand, is composed of a more delicate tissue known as squamous epithelium. Barrett's esophagus occurs when the regurgitated stomach acid chronically burns the tender lining of the esophagus, and the body goes into defense mode trying to protect the esophagus from ensuing danger. It does so by replacing the acid-destroyed squamous cells in the lining of the esophagus with a special type of acid-resistant columnar epithelium similar to that which lines the stomach and intestine. This change is called metaplasia.

Ideally, that new lining of columnar epithelium cells similar to those protecting the stomach should also protect the esophagus from being burned. It must do this to some extent because often the symptoms of GERD actually lessen or disappear completely when someone has Barrett's esophagus. But ironically, something alarming also takes place in the foreign territory of the esophagus: The displaced or metaplastic columnar epithelium now covering parts of the esophagus becomes premalignant. Researchers still don't understand just why this happens. According to H. Worth Boyce, Jr., M.D., director of the Joy McCann Culverhouse Center for Swallowing Disorders at the University of South Florida in Tampa, "Patients with adenocarcinoma developing in the esophagus have an associated columnar-lined esophagus in nearly all cases."

Who Is Most Prone to Developing Barrett's Esophagus?

Barrett's esophagus is three times more common in men than women, especially Caucasian men age fifty and over. It is sometimes, although rarely, found in children, but those patients tend to have another serious disorder as well such as cystic fibrosis, neurological impairment, mental retardation, or a hiatal hernia.

African Americans are less likely to have Barrett's esophagus or even GERD, for that matter. A recent study done at the Arizona Health Sciences Center and Tucson Veteran Affairs Medical Center revealed that the prevalence of Barrett's esophagus in Hispanic patients was similar to that in Caucasian patients.

Barrett's Esophagus May Be Present Without Heartburn or Other Symptoms

Don't think you couldn't possibly have Barrett's esophagus because you don't suffer from heartburn or because your heartburn has gone away since you started taking over-the-counter medications. You don't need to have heartburn to develop Barrett's esophagus. Remember that heartburn is merely one of many symptoms of gastroesophageal reflux disease. In some people, there may only be a slight hoarseness or a chronic cough to alert them that something might be wrong. But as much as a third of those suffering from Barrett's esophagus have few if any symptoms. This unfortunately keeps those individuals from seeing their physician, which probably accounts for the alarming amount of destruction created by BE by the time people do begin to have symptoms. According to *Current Medical Diagnosis & Treatment 1999*, "Over 90% of individuals with Barrett's esophagus in the general population do not seek medical attention and go unrecognized."[9]

How Barrett's Esophagus Is Diagnosed

The best way for a gastroenterologist to determine if you have Barrett's esophagus is to perform what's called an upper gastrointestinal endoscopy (esophagoscopy with biopsy).

Although it's an invasive procedure, it's relatively mild with little, if any, discomfort.

Your throat will be sprayed with an anesthetic to numb the area and relax the gag reflex and you'll be given sedation through an I.V., although you will remain aware and able to follow instructions (conscious sedation). Then an extremely thin, flexible, lighted tube called an endoscope is inserted into your mouth, down your throat, and into your esophagus. A miniature videocamera at the end of the scope casts a view of the entire surface area of your esophagus on a screen for the doctor to see. It will reveal any columnar-appearing esophageal mucosa (a sign of BE). The gastroenterologist also may take tiny tissue samples (biopsies) of suspicious areas at this time. The entire procedure usually takes less than fifteen minutes, and you can leave the office immediately afterward and do your normal activities. Because of the sedation, you need to avoid driving, however, or any other potentially dangerous physical activity for twenty-four hours.

How Barrett's Esophagus Is Treated

At this writing, there is no definitive medical or surgical way to reverse Barrett's esophagus once it exists, although various avenues may be considered to slow and manage the gastroesophageal reflux. Methods to remove BE cells and allow for regrowth of normal esophageal cells are currently being evaluated.

MEDICATIONS

Although there are no drugs available to eradicate Barrett's esophagus, there are many medications such as antacids, H_2 blockers, and proton pump inhibitors that can relieve symptoms of GERD. (You'll read more about these medications in Chapter 5.) The proton pump inhibitors, Prilosec, Prevacid, Nexium, Protonix, and Aciphex, which prevent acid from forming in the stomach, seem to slow the progress of Barrett's esophagus.

Prilosec is expected to be available without a prescription in 2002, but this may be a double-edged sword. There is a great concern voiced by many gastroenterologists that as the PPIs become available over-the-counter, people will pop these pills to control their heartburn and, satisfied with the relief they get, fail to see a doctor to be screened for Barrett's esophagus.

"I'm not so sure it's such a good idea to make these medications OTC," said retired Tampa gastroenterologist Joel Fyvolent. "They can mask far more serious symptoms."

SURGERY

In a surgical procedure called an esophagectomy, the surgeon removes a section of the diseased esophagus. This may be an option in specific cases, but it is a most difficult operation from which to recover and has an uncertain outcome. It also causes major lifestyle changes and has the potential for continuing medical problems.

PHOTODYNAMIC THERAPY[10]

In the past few years, selected physicians around the world have been utilizing a technique called photodynamic therapy (PDT) to try to eradicate Barrett's esophagus. This type of treatment has been FDA approved for certain lung cancers and late-stage esophageal cancers. It is in clinical trials for cancers of the head, neck, breast, bladder, skin, and brain. At this writing, PDT has not yet been approved by the Food and Drug Administration for use in treating Barrett's esophagus and is considered to be investigational.

In treating Barrett's esophagus, the aim of photodynamic therapy is to prevent the premalignant cells from becoming cancerous. It is less invasive and less expensive than surgery. A patient is injected in a vein with a special drug called

Photofrin that makes tissues highly sensitive to light. Cells that are cancerous or even precancerous absorb the drug. Forty-eight hours after the injection, the patient is sedated and an endoscope is inserted into the esophagus. A deflated balloon is passed into the esophagus, positioned, and then inflated to keep the folds of the esophagus open when the light beam is activated. A special type of laser probe, called a cylindrical diffuser, is inserted inside the balloon and activated. A special laser delivers light to the cylindrical diffuser. When the drug retained in the cells is exposed to this laser light, the drug produces a chemical that kills the abnormal cells.

After another forty-eight hours, the effect on the premalignant columnar-lined tissues in the esophagus is apparent. The exudate (leftover burned materials) can be seen. Thermal ablation by a different laser or electrothermal probe is used for any last remaining bits of Barrett's tissue found during follow-up endoscopy, usually at three months or later.

Drs. Bergein Overholt and Masoud Panjehpour of the Thompson Cancer Survival Center in Knoxville are pioneers in using the PDT procedure for Barrett's esophaghus and initiated the multi-center randomized PDT study. Dr. Overholt is encouraged by the results thus far. He has been working with PDT for 11 years and has treated more than 390 patients.

Our research indicates that patient outcomes, when defined as lower morbidity [incidence of a disease], mortality, and cost, are improved by using PDT as the treatment for Barrett's dysplasia. By treating Barrett's esophagus before it becomes cancerous, we have the potential to decrease the number of Barrett's patients later diagnosed with esophageal cancer.

Drs. Overholt and Panjehpour have recently begun trials using Levulan (aminolevulinic acid, or ALA) in PDT for patients with no dysplasia, as well as low- and high-grade dysplasia. A specially developed cylindrical balloon is inflated within the esophagus and used to direct the laser light to the Barrett's tissue. The balloon helps to deliver the light to the Barrett's esophagus as well as to minimize the damage to surrounding healthy tissue. Again, the possibility of destroying the Barrett's tissue in earlier stages hopefully will further reduce the likelihood of these patients later developing esophageal cancer. These trials are ongoing at Thompson Cancer Survival Center

Photodynamic therapy is not without its unpleasant side effects, however. Since the drug is taken up by all of the cells in the body, the same properties that cause the reaction with the laser light also cause a reaction to sunlight. Patients under treatment with the Photofrin drug have severe skin photosensitivity for about thirty days after treatment and must stay completely covered (including long sleeves, long pants, hat, ski mask, sunglasses, and gloves) or indoors to avoid a severe sunburn. Photosensitivity is much less profound in the ALA treatments. In these patients, photosensitivity lasts only 48–72 hours since the Levulan drug clears the body more rapidly. Also, with both drugs, some patients may feel some nausea after the procedure and will not be too inclined to eat for a time. Obviously, there is swelling and tightness in the chest, making it uncomfortable to swallow. Patients also may carry a low-grade fever, mid-chest pain, or experience shortness of breath.

Early experience with PDT produced strictures (narrowing of the esophagus) in over 50 percent of patients, but this complication has recently decreased to about 25 percent that may require dilation. Nevertheless, PDT sounds promising and it is hoped that future results will prove successful in furthering photodynamic therapy as an accepted treatment for eradicating Barrett's esophagus before it can turn into a full blown case of esophageal cancer.

LONG-TERM CARE

If it is determined that you do have Barrett's esophagus, you need to accept the fact that you will require medical care for the rest of your life. Your physician will want you to return regularly for additional endoscopes and biopsies to be sure that a malignancy doesn't exist. Don't put off those regular appointments. Your life may depend on them.

Esophageal Cancer

Illness is the doctor to whom we pay the most heed;
to kindness, to knowledge, we make promises only;
to pain we obey.

—MARCEL PROUST

ESOPHAGEAL ADENOCARCINOMA is what the physicians call it. Most laypeople call it cancer of the esophagus. For thousands, this most aggressive disease may be the end result of long-term suffering from chronic "simple" heartburn problems. For reasons unknown to physicians and researchers, the frequency of esophageal adenocarcinoma in the United States and Western Europe is increasing dramatically. It is virtually always associated with Barrett's esophagus except in extremely rare cases.

According to the American Cancer Society, more than 12,500 new cases are diagnosed each year, primarily among white males age fifty and over. "In 1975, less than 10 percent of the esophageal cancers were adenocarcinoma," said H. Worth Boyce, Jr., M.D. "Now 75 percent of them are and we don't know why, other than their association with Barrett's esophagus." The National Institutes of Health also expressed concern. "The risk of esophageal cancer is growing; over the past 20 years the incidence rate has increased 14.8

percent."[11] At this growing rate, esophageal adenocarcinoma will soon become a common form of cancer.

The Symptoms of Esophageal Adenocarcinoma

Unfortunately, the symptoms of esophageal cancer often don't show up until the disease is fairly severe and has spread to the surrounding lymph nodes or to other areas of the body. The first symptom that usually brings someone to see the doctor is difficulty swallowing.

Other presenting symptoms may include a sensation of fullness or a burning feeling in the throat. Some people choke easily on their food or actually vomit it up. There also may be coughing, an unexplained hoarseness, or even pain.

It's important to remember, however, that many of these symptoms could also be caused by other disorders, some of which are far less serious than esophageal adenocarcinoma. Nevertheless, you should never try to self-diagnose or just assume that your symptoms are really caused by something minor. Denial can be deadly. Always see your physician for a correct diagnosis—even if you are a doctor yourself.

What Causes Esophageal Adenocarcinoma?

A 1999 study by Swedish researchers headed by Jesper Lagergren, M.D., of the Karolinski Institute in Stockholm, found that the risk of esophageal cancer was almost eight times as high in those who suffered from weekly heartburn and gastroesophageal reflux disease when compared with nonsufferers. Those who experienced nocturnal reflux (waking up with heartburn or a bitter taste in the mouth) were associated with a risk of developing esophageal cancer that was eleven times as high as the control group. According to the study, the longer these various symptoms persist, the higher the risk of cancer, especially if Barrett's esophagus has developed.[12]

But at least a quarter of those individuals diagnosed with

Barrett's esophagus have few, if any, symptoms of reflux. Therefore, they often aren't aware of having any type of medical problem. Unfortunately, it isn't until they begin to develop difficulty swallowing or experience any of the other more serious complications that these patients usually seek medical care.

What Happens When a Cancer Grows in the Esophagus

Small tumors in the esophagus usually aren't particularly noticed because they seldom create any symptoms. It's only when the tumor begins to grow that the person feels something uncomfortable. There may be difficulty or pain swallowing. Remember that the average esophagus is only ten inches long and about three-quarters of an inch in width. That's about the size of a nickel or quarter. Therefore, it's no surprise that when a tumor starts growing even slightly larger it creates a noticeable blockage. Solid food, especially meats and bread, begin to stick in the throat. Then even soft foods like custard as well as liquids become difficult to swallow. The individual begins to lose significant weight.

How Esophageal Adenocarcinoma Is Diagnosed

Although blood work and X rays usually are performed to determine the extent of the problem, the diagnosis of esophageal adenocarcinoma is usually made after an endoscopy and biopsy. Then the tumor is staged in order to determine how far the disease has progressed and what course of action may be taken. If the cancer has already metastasized or spread to other parts of the body, the options become more limited. As with most cancers, however, the five-year survival rate for those whose esophageal adenocarcinomas are detected early is far better than those whose malignancies are discovered after they have spread.

What Is the Treatment for
Esophageal Adenocarcinoma?

Esophageal adenocarcinoma is a nasty disease with a poor survival rate. Because it usually is diagnosed only after the symptoms are noticeable and become intolerable, the disease often is quite advanced. Unfortunately, unless esophageal adenocarcinoma is found in its earliest stages, the prognosis usually is poor. Determining a way to continue nutrition as well as preventing pneumonia are major problems.

Only 12 percent of patients newly diagnosed with esophageal adenocarcinoma survive five or more years. That's why it's so important for individuals diagnosed with Barrett's esophagus to have regular annual endoscopies in order to be certain that the premalignant cells haven't changed to become malignant. That's also why it's important for you to take even mild, but chronic heartburn and reflux seriously.

DILATION AND STENT PLACEMENT

To help the patient swallow more easily, a brief procedure called dilation opens the narrowing walls of the esophagus and keeps them open in order to permit fluids and soft foods to pass through. With the patient sedated, the gastroenterologist gently inserts a dilator, a plastic or water-filled balloon device, into the esophagus. This dilator stretches the narrowed segment to keep the esophagus open; however, the tumor often narrows the esophagus in a short time.

Since dilation typically produces short-term relief, the use of a stent or prosthesis often proves to be the best therapy. A stent is a plastic or metal mesh cylinder that expands after insertion to provide a more permanent opening through the cancer. The patient is then much better able to swallow and maintain nutrition.

PHOTODYNAMIC THERAPY

A photosensitizing drug is given intravenously. (PDT is described earlier in this chapter.) It then collects in the tumor, which causes a chemical reaction between the drug and laser light, cutting the oxygen supply to the cells of the tumor. In early stages of a noninvasive cancer, the tumor is destroyed. In cases where the the tumor is obstructing the esophagus, much of the tumor is debulked (reduced in size), making swallowing more comfortable for the patient.

SURGERY

Surgery (sometimes followed by radiation) to reduce the size of the tumor or to resect the esophagus to make it easier for the person to eat may be done. Unfortunately, there is only a 25 to 50 percent three-year survival rate. "By the time patients undergo attempted curative resection, more than 80 percent of patients have widespread metastases to bone marrow."[13] The success of surgery for cure is directly related to the extent of cancer growth. Early diagnosis is the key.

With the drastic increase of esophageal adenocarcinoma, not only in the United States but also throughout Western Europe, researchers are working to discover new or more effective treatments to extend the survival rates for those with the disease.

For more information about esophageal adenocarcinoma, contact the National Cancer Institute at 1-800-422-6237. The call is free, and the staff can talk with you in either English or Spanish.

Chapter Four

Seeking Proper Medical Care

When to Go to the Doctor

YOU'VE BEEN experiencing heartburn and symptoms of GERD for at least a month or two. You've been taking over-the-counter medications that seem to help for a few hours, but then you feel discomfort again. Or you wake during the night with a bad taste in your mouth, and you always seem to be hoarse in the morning.

Should you see a doctor with these symptoms? And if so, who? With so many different medical specialties, what type of physician treats heartburn? What about hoarseness? Or laryngitis? You feel as though it would just be easier to throw a dart at some doctor dart board and see where it lands.

When You Should Seek Medical Help

Most physicians who treat people with GERD say that these patients wait too long before they seek help, self-medicating themselves with a variety of over-the-counter medications or herbal preparations for heartburn and other symptoms of GERD, rather than going to see a doctor. In my survey of more than a dozen people with GERD, all but one waited one or more years until the pain grew almost unbearable before seeking treatment.

One respondent, my cousin Wayne Grody, a physician himself, suffered from heartburn for ten to fifteen years and didn't seek medical help until "my symptoms changed to angina-like chest pains and I thought I was having a heart attack."

Gordon Lenci, owner of a B and B in New England, said, "I was diagnosed with a hiatal hernia and paid no attention to it for twelve to fourteen years. Then I got heavy chest pains. After numerous tests—stress test, endoscopy, colonoscopy, etc.—the doctor prescribed Prilosec. The symptoms virtually disappeared. I stopped taking the medication recently and now have indigestion only when I eat the wrong foods."

A woman who had suffered from GERD since her pregnancy waited eight years before finally deciding to see a physician.

GERD is a chronic disease. It won't get better by waiting and just hoping it will go away on its own. What's more, the symptoms of GERD can mask serious and even potentially fatal problems, as you read in Chapter 3. Delay can be deadly.

Marvin Schuster, M.D., professor of medicine and psychiatry at the Johns Hopkins University School of Medicine and director of the Division of Digestive Diseases at the Johns Hopkins Bayview Medical Center, advises, "You should see a doctor if your symptoms occur more than three times a week or if you're awakened at night by symptoms. Also see your doctor at the slightest hint of having food sticking in your throat, aspirating food, or choking at night."

H. Worth Boyce, Jr., M.D., described "alarm symptoms" that should get you up off your chair and to the telephone, calling for an immediate medical appointment.

- difficulty swallowing

- weight loss

- symptoms of anemia (such as extreme fatigue, light-headedness, or pallor)

- bleeding

- pain (that is constant, long in duration, felt in the chest and back and doesn't respond to antacids or food; it may mean the tumor has metastasized to the nerve endings)

What Type of Doctor Should You See?

Depending on your type of insurance coverage, you may have little choice of what type of doctor to see initially. Your only option may be your primary care physician, who should in turn refer you to a specialist when necessary.

But with managed care in place, it often is difficult to get that referral to a specialist. If your primary care physician doesn't know what is wrong, or if his or her suggestions do not ease your symptoms, then insist on a referral to a specialist.

Sometimes it isn't the physician who interferes with the patient's opportunity to see a specialist; it's the insurance company. A 1999 survey conducted for the Kaiser Family Foundation (a nonprofit health research group) with the Harvard School of Public Health revealed that 42 percent of the 1,053 physicians surveyed said they had encountered a denial of diagnostic tests or procedures by their patients' insurance plans at least once a month or even once a week. Overall, 77 percent of the doctors surveyed said that managed care had decreased the ability of patients to get the tests and treatments they need, while 86 percent said it had decreased the ability of patients to see medical specialists.

Later in this chapter I list some ways you as a layperson can help your doctor force the issue so you can see a specialist when necessary. Meanwhile, it's important for you to know who these specialists are and which ones to see when.

Internists

Your first stop probably will be your internist. With many medical insurance plans, the internist is your assigned medical insurance gatekeeper. But don't confuse an internist with an intern. An internist is a specialist who is trained in the essentials of primary care internal medicine, including disease prevention, wellness, substance abuse, mental health, and treatment of common problems of the eyes, ears, skin, nervous system, and reproductive organs.

An intern, on the other hand, is a doctor in the first year of training after graduating from medical school. ("Intern" is an older term; the more usual terminology today is "resident," regardless if it's the physician's first, second, or third year of training.)

While the internist can treat you for heartburn, he or she will probably want to refer you to a specialist if you have multiple symptoms of GERD or if your reflux symptoms are severe. The type of specialist you'll be sent to will depend on your presenting symptoms—heartburn, difficulty swallowing, chronic sore throat or hoarseness, chronic cough, belching, or actual regurgitation.

Family Practitioners

A family doctor or family practitioner or GP (general practitioner) provides medical care to everyone in the family, from infants to the elderly. A family practitioner or GP may serve in the same gatekeeping capacity as an internist, although because the family practitioner is trained in pediatrics, obstetrics, and other family needs, there is less focus on specialties such as gastroenterology.

Pediatricians

Pediatricians specialize in the care, development, and treatment of children from newborn to eighteen years of age, although some pediatricians see their regular patients up to age twenty-one. (One of my daughters clung to her pediatrician longer than she did her teddy bear.)

While most pediatricians use positioning and dietary changes to treat infants with GERD (see Chapter 2), they may refer the patient to a pediatric gastroenterologist if the GERD is severe.

Otolaryngologists

An otolaryngologist (more popularly known as an ENT, meaning ear, nose, and throat) is a medical specialist who cares for people with diseases and disorders affecting the ears, respiratory and upper alimentary systems, and related structures, and the head and neck in general. You may be referred to this type of physician if you suffer from chronic hoarseness or chronic laryngitis.

Allergists and Immunologists

Allergists and immunologists specialize in the diagnosis and treatment of allergies. These physicians treat people who suffer from asthma, a disease often found in those with GERD. (See Chapter 3 for more information on the connection between asthma and gastroesophageal reflux disease.)

Gastroenterologists

A gastroenterologist specializes in the function and disorders of the digestive tract, which includes the esophagus, stomach, intestines, and related organs of the gastrointestinal tract. Gastroenterologists probably have the most experience performing endoscopies for GERD. Most of those who perform endoscopy are members of the American Society for Gastrointestinal Endoscopy.

Pediatric Gastroenterologists

A pediatric gastroenterologist has taken additional training in pediatrics in order to be able to diagnose and treat infants and children. This pediatric age group is not just "little adults." The esophagus is smaller in children. The instruments must be smaller and the person doing the endoscopy needs to have experience working with a pediatric population.

Pulmonologists

Pulmonologists have received extra training in dealing with the function and disorders of the lungs. If you have developed aspiration pneumonia from breathing in refluxed material as you sleep, you probably will be referred to this specialist.

Gastrointestinal Endoscopic Surgeons

Most people with GERD respond well to both lifestyle modifications and medication. Some patients, however, require surgery to successfully treat their GERD. (See Chapter 5 for more information on the type of surgery available when you have severe GERD.) The most common type of surgery performed today is the laparoscopic Nissen fundoplication.

Surgeons who perform this type of surgery are specially

trained to use the laparoscope. Many of them belong to the Society of American Gastrointestinal Endoscopic Surgeons.

How to Find the Right Doctor for You

Locating a physician to take care of you used to be strictly a personal choice. You'd check with friends, relatives, business associates, or even the local medical association. When the same name kept popping up, you'd call and make an appointment to see that physician.

Now, with managed care dictating what doctors are available for you, it's more difficult in many ways. You might not recognize a single name on the list of providers. What's worse, no one you talk to recognizes any of them either. But don't give up. You can make an educated decision. It just takes more time. And sometimes you may need to see more than one physician before you find a good match.

- Ask friends who are health care professionals to help you select a primary care physician. Listen to what they say (and don't say).

- Don't choose a doctor because the office is nearby or you've heard the name somewhere. Your primary care doctor is the key to opening doors to the proper specialist.

- Get to know the doctor's office staff by name. Not only will they be able to work you in when you really need to see the doctor, but these individuals also are often the ones who know how to work the system when it comes to insurance issues.

- Don't expect your doctor to be a mind reader. If you want to know everything—good and bad—about your disease, treatment, and side effects, then say so. Some people don't want to have too much information and just trust the doctor to make the decisions. But if you're like I am and want to know it all, ask the doctor to explain in more detail. If you don't understand, ask him or her to translate the medical jargon into plain old English.

- Realize that your doctor is pressed for time and don't waste it. Have your questions written down so you don't forget. But if you don't understand the answer, ask if there is a nurse in the office who can spend more time with you.

- Ask your physician which medications, tests, or procedures he or she would suggest regardless if your insurance covers it or not. You may decide to pay for it yourself if you can't convince the insurance company to do so.

- If your "gatekeeper" won't open the gate for you to see a specialist or have specific diagnostic tests or treatment, find another who will, even if you have to pay for it yourself. Many managed care plans pay bonuses to primary care physicians who spend less money on specialists for patient care. (It's like having your sink repaired by a plumber who gets paid more for doing less work.) It's your body; you need to be your own advocate.

- Don't think only in terms of people with an M.D. after their name. Six percent of all U.S. physicians are D.O.'s (doctors of osteopathic medicine). According to John P. Sevastos, past president of the American Osteopathic Association, "D.O.'s have essentially the same qualifications, medical education, internship, licensure, and specialties as M.D.'s. They are equal with M.D.'s under the laws of all fifty states, serve as commissioned officers in the medical corps of all armed forces, plus the Veterans Administration and Public Health Service.

And they are recognized as physicians by the AMA. Moreover, 31 percent of the profession is board certified in a full range of medical specialties, including surgery, anesthesiology, emergency medicine, psychiatry, obstetrics, pediatrics, radiology, and others." To find a D.O. in your area, call the American Osteopathic Association at 1-800-621-1773 or go to their Web site at www.aoa_net.org.

- Feel comfortable with the physician you select. Patients with GERD have a chronic disease. That means you're going to spend a long time interacting with this individual. Studies have shown that when patients establish a rapport with their physician, they tend to be more compliant (follow instructions) and do better with their disease. Communication is the key to establishing a good relationship.

- Learn all you can about your disease. It's easier for physicians to help you when you're up to speed on the most recent developments pertaining to the treatment and long-term effects of your disease. You can't become a partner in your health care unless you fully understand what's happening to your body.

How to Handle Insurance Issues

What can you do if your insurance plan denies your seeing a specialist or having diagnostic tests?

Your internist or family physician may likely recommend that you see a specialist to undergo specific diagnostic tests for your symptoms of GERD. Then he or she may add, "But your insurance won't cover it."

What can you do? How can David fight the Goliath of managed care big business? Here are some suggestions to help you get the health care, including diagnosis and proper treatment, you need and deserve.[1]

- If you are selecting a health plan and choosing between various HMO or PPO plans, don't necessarily pick the cheapest one. It could be a costly mistake in terms of your health.

- Read every bit of material you are sent by your managed care plan. Most of us just stick the envelope in a desk drawer and forget about it. Ask about parts you don't understand.

- If your health insurance is obtained through your work, tell the person in charge of human resources if you're not happy with the service you're getting. Your complaint may be the final straw that convinces your boss it's time for a change.

- Go over your primary physician's head, if necessary, and challenge the HMO yourself. Ask for the supervisor (everyone has one). Don't take no for an answer. The informed patient is a threat to the managed care industry. If your primary care physician is on your side, so much the better. It's (sometimes) a winning combination.

- If you're not satisfied with the treatment you receive from your managed care organization, talk about it to others. You may not be the only unhappy subscriber. Remember, for them it's a business, and too many lost subscribers can affect their profits. For you, it's your life. That makes it worth fighting for.

- Write to your state legislator or Congress representatives or contact the media if you feel you're not getting proper health care from your managed care organization.

Can it be done? Can you overturn the original decision made by your health insurance company? Yes. It's been done successfully more often than you might think. Good luck!

Chapter Five

What Treatment Is Available

Lifestyle Changes That Often Alleviate Symptoms

Happy is said to be the family which can eat onions together.

—CHARLES DUDLEY WARNER

MY CHILDHOOD summers were spent at Lake Okoboji in northwestern Iowa. My paternal grandparents had a large cottage with ample room for their four adult children and the spouses and a large sleeping porch for the ever-growing brood of grandchildren, of which I was the youngest until the last few years we vacationed there.

After lunch, which was the large main meal served at "Sunny Side," my grandfather would go into the common room and take a nap on the daybed, which was tucked away in a corner. We, the grandkids, waited anxiously for him to wake up and go fishing because the slant of the daybed allowed the coins in his pocket to slip out and fall between the cushions as he slept. Then it was our turn to go fishing for as much change as we could retrieve before we were pushed aside by the older cousins.

But what I remember as vividly as the coin collecting was that my grandfather always woke up complaining that the noon meal had given him indigestion and that "no man should have to swallow his meal twice."

At the time, I didn't give his comment much thought, other than that it seemed a funny thing to say. Now, as an adult, I wonder if my grandfather suffered from gastroesophageal reflux disease. If so, his heavy noon meal and after-lunch nap no doubt made his symptoms even worse.

Today, most knowledgeable physicians urge their patients who seem to be suffering from GERD to consider making lifestyle modifications. If the individuals are willing to carry out these changes and do so faithfully and most of the symptoms disappear or are minimized, it's a pretty good chance that it is GERD.

Making these lifestyle changes isn't always easy. We humans are creatures of habit, and change is difficult. You probably know this from experience if you've tried to stay on a diet to lose weight, tackle an exercise program, or even rearrange your closet and keep reaching for something that's now in a new place.

Gastroesophageal reflux disease, however, is a chronic disease, so these lifestyle changes you need to make can't be a sometime thing. The modifications must become a permanent way of life. But lasting lifestyle changes may be difficult to accomplish, as they require discipline and persistence. On the plus side, however, they also are, for the most part, free and have no harmful side effects.

Think Small When It Comes to the Size of Your Meals

Most of us eat too much, especially for dinner. It used to be that we ate massive meals only at holidays like Thanksgiving, Christmas, Hanukkah, Passover, or Easter. Now the "all you can eat" philosophy has permeated not only our kitchens but also our restaurants and fast food eateries. A sixteen-ounce steak or triple cheeseburger has become the norm, adding inches to our waistlines and intensifying the symptoms of heartburn and GERD.

So think small when you sit down to a meal. Eating smaller, more frequent meals reduces the pressure on the LES, making it less likely that the contents of your stomach will reflux into your esophagus and mouth. If you must eat a large meal, make it at noon rather than in the evening with bedtime only a few hours away. In fact, try to avoid eating anything two to three hours before going to bed.

There are a number of foods that you also should avoid when you have GERD, but because it's so important to become aware of what they are, these foods are mentioned in a separate section of this chapter. Be sure to read that section carefully so you know which foods and beverages to avoid when you suffer from heartburn and GERD.

Don't Recline After You Dine

You shouldn't lie down for at least two to three hours after eating. That gives the contents of your stomach a chance to be broken up and partially digested and to begin to pass into the small intestine. This delay between eating and lying down will help to reduce the possibility of reflux. If my grandfather had had this information, he might have enjoyed his noon meal more.

Heads Up When You Sleep

Most of us sleep in a horizontal position. When you have GERD, however, that position allows gravity to work against you, not only putting pressure on the LES, which permits reflux to take place, but also letting the gastric acid to remain in your esophagus for too long a period of time. For this reason, experts suggest that you raise the head of your bed by six inches so your esophagus is well above your stomach.

Sleeping on two or more pillows won't help the situation, though. Pillows tend to shift as you sleep. Also, you tend to scrunch down, compressing your stomach and creating more pressure on the lower esophageal sphincter. Instead, try placing a six-inch block or bricks under each leg at the head of your bed. That will keep your head (and, unfortunately, that of your sleep partner, as well) elevated to the proper height so stomach acid can't back up into your esophagus. Blocks such as these can be purchased in health supply stores or ordered through various health care catalogs. Note: If you make them yourself, be sure they are stable and skid-proof. You also can use a coffee can filled with sand.

You also can use a firm foam wedge that fits under the bottom sheet "from butt to head," as one doctor expressed it. This type of product, one of which is called Bedge, can be purchased in medical supply stores or in your local pharmacy and may be found in many health care catalogs. For information on the Bedge, call 619-340-3813.

Clinicians suggest that you sleep on your left side, if possible, as sleeping on your right side allows stomach acid to seep more easily into the esophagus, causing nocturnal reflux. This type of reflux causes great harm to your esophagus because when we sleep the flow of saliva is reduced so there is less saliva to dilute the refluxed material. There also is more chance for the acid gastric contents to be inhaled into our lungs as we sleep, causing aspiration pneumonia.

Stop Smoking

Every physician I interviewed for this book said the most important message to relay to my readers is: "Stop smoking!"

The cigarette smoke irritates the delicate lining of the digestive tract, which makes the tissue even more vulnerable to irritation when bathed by refluxed stomach acid. "Smoking increases air swallowing, belching, and relaxes the lower esophageal sphincter that protects your esophagus from the backwash of stomach contents," said Tampa allergy and immunology specialist Richard F. Lockey, M.D. And, according to Henry D. Janowitz, M.D., even "sucking a cigar all day long can lead to air swallowing, which increases stomach pressure and favors reflux." What's more, nicotine reduces the flow of saliva and increases stomach acid, both of which aggravate reflux.

There are many products available to help you stop smoking. Ask your physician for suggestions as to which one would be most beneficial to you. Heartburn and gastric reflux are just two of the medical problems made more critical by nicotine. Heart disease, cancer (of the esophagus, lung, bladder, pancreas, tongue, larynx, etc.), and emphysema are others—and the list goes on. Follow the advice of all physicians and stop smoking.

Avoid Bending Over

When you bend over, you put additional pressure on your stomach, which forces stomach acid to back up into the esophagus. Instead, squat, with your knees bent, when you pick up things (it's also better for your back).

Avoid Wearing Tight Clothing

You may ask what a particular clothing style has to do with reducing heartburn and GERD. Actually, it has a great deal to do with it. Tight clothing such as form-fitting jeans, snug belts, stiff waist-length jackets, and firm undergarments (that used to be called "waist cinchers," "girdles," and "minimizers") put added pressure on the digestive tract, which increases the potential for heartburn and GERD. It makes you wonder if medieval knights in full armor suffered from GERD.

This knowledge that constrictive clothing can trigger digestive ailments is hardly new. In 1866, an English physician named Thomas King Chambers wrote a book called *The Indigestions or Diseases of the Digestive Organs Functionally Treated.* In it he wrote of the medical problems inherent in "tight-lacing" He wrote, "The section of the waist seemed to admit of no room for anything else at all. . . . The organ which suffers most is the unresisting stomach, which is dragged and pushed out of all form during the continuance of this packing process." Dr. Chambers performed seemingly wondrous cures when he advised his female patients to "remove the obnoxious stays."

Although women no longer wear corsets with stays, many of us still "lace" ourselves into tight fitting clothes or wrap belts a size too small around our waists and then wonder why our heartburn seems worse.

Lose Weight

As described earlier, people who lose weight are often amazed that it also minimizes their symptoms of heartburn and GERD. But it makes sense if you think about it. When you lose weight, fat deposits inside your abdomen are reduced as well as on the outside where people notice it. This decreases the pressure from within the stomach against the lower esophageal sphincter. When there is less pressure buildup, the valve is less likely to leak acid back up into the esophagus.

A periodontist I interviewed for this book called me to say, "I can't be a subject for your book anymore. I've lost twenty-two pounds and I don't seem to have heartburn or GERD anymore, or at least the symptoms aren't bad anymore."

Excess weight is involved in creating problems in many other medical conditions, such as heart disease, high blood pressure, many forms of cancer, adult onset diabetes, arthritis, and respiratory problems. If you've been trying to lose weight, here's another reason why you should keep at it. Lose pounds and keep heartburn and GERD at bay.

Exercise

Closely related to helping you lose weight, exercise also can modify the effects of heartburn and GERD. Exercise reduces stress and helps you to feel good about yourself, which in turn makes it more likely that you'll quit smoking and begin to eat a more healthy diet.

However, the type of exercise you engage in could also bring on symptoms of heartburn and GERD. In a study conducted by Dr. Donald Castell and others, running caused more reflux than did other forms of exercise, a finding that will make many joggers nod their heads in agreement. In this study, weight lifting and bicycling were the least likely to trigger heartburn or actual regurgitation.

For many people, walking seems to be the choice exercise. You already know how to do it, and there's no age limitation. Walking requires no special clothes (other than comfortable shoes), no partner, and no specific place you need to travel to in order to engage in it. What's more, just a half hour of brisk walking daily can help you lose fifteen pounds in one year. What constitutes a brisk walk? Walking fast enough that you're breathing hard, but not so fast that you're gasping when you try to speak. *Prevention* magazine has long been a proponent of walking as an exercise and each issue seems to have at least one article highlighting walking. If you can't picture walking as a legitimate form of exercise, look up some back issues. They'll change your mind.

Note: Always check with your physician before starting an exercise program. If you feel pain, stop immediately. Heartburn often feels like chest pains, but never try to make your own diagnosis. See a trained medical professional. Better safe than sorry.

Recommended Lifestyle Modifications for GERD*

- Eat small meals

- Choose low-fat foods

- Reduce intake of chocolate, carminatives (peppermint or spearmint), and alcohol

- Limit consumption of beverages containing caffeine

- Limit consumption of carbonated beverages

- Stop cigarette smoking

- Suck hard candies or chew gum to increase saliva

- Don't lie down for 2 to 3 hours after eating

- Sleep with the head of the bed elevated 6 inches

- Wear loose-fitting clothing

- Take an OTC H$_2$-receptor antagonist or antacid as needed for symptoms.

*Reprinted with permission from Practical Gastroenterology, *February 1999.*

Foods to Avoid

For a bad night,
a mattress of wine.

—SPANISH PROVERB

YOU HAVE only to watch television for a few nights to see a constant parade of commercials assuring viewers that they can eat anything they want without suffering from heartburn or GERD just by taking a particular pill or liquid either before or after eating. And so we flock like lemmings to the drugstore or supermarket to buy that specific product in hopes of finding our gastronomic utopia: the ability to eat whatever we want without any consequences. Almost 40 million Americans take some type of over-the-counter antacid or H$_2$-receptor antagonist at least twice a week to make their heartburn and other acid reflux symptoms go away. No wonder the antacid business is a $3 billion industry.

Yet as each of us is unique, one person's meat truly is another person's poison. Actually, the name of this section should have been "Foods You *Might* Need to Avoid"—because while there are specific foods that tend to cause heartburn and GERD symptoms for many people, they may not be triggers for you. *Don't arbitrarily drop all these listed foods from your diet just because they're mentioned here.*

Instead, begin to keep a detection diary (described later in this section) to see what foods trigger pain and discomfort for you. You may be surprised to discover that what bothers your spouse, friend, or coworker gives you no problem at all.

How Foods Trigger GERD

There are three different ways food acts as a trigger for heartburn and other symptoms of GERD. What we eat or drink can:

- irritate or burn the delicate tissues of the esophageal wall going down or when the bolus mixed with stomach acid is regurgitated

- slow down peristalsis so the food remains in the stomach longer, allowing more chance for reflux

- weaken or relax the lower esophageal sphincter so the food mixed with acid begins to reflux into the esophagus and throat

Foods That Are Common Triggers

CITRUS

It doesn't matter if you eat an orange or squeeze it for juice. The acidity in oranges, as well as in grapefruit and lemons, irritates the esophagus and can trigger reflux. People with a history of heartburn or other symptoms of GERD who gulp down a glass of orange juice on an empty stomach as they dash out the door for work can vouch for this.

CAFFEINE-CONTAINING BEVERAGES

This includes not only coffee (both decaffeinated *and* regular) but also tea (especially with mint), cocoa, and soft drinks with caffeine, such as colas.

CHOCOLATE

Chocolate is a common trigger for many people with heartburn and other symptoms of GERD. Obviously, drinking coffee with chocolate makes it even worse, and when you add whipping cream, it can become a painful pastime.

PEPPERMINT

For years people have followed the old wives' tale that tells you to take a peppermint to "settle" your stomach. But peppermint is a common trigger for both heartburn and many of the other symptoms of GERD. It's surprising, then, that so many of the finest hotels and B and B's continue to place chocolate-covered peppermints on guests' pillows, with a note wishing them to "sleep well."

FATTY FOODS

Fatty foods such as fried foods, hot dogs, bacon, and the like weaken or reduce the pressure in the lower esophageal sphincter and tend to promote reflux.

DAIRY PRODUCTS

Cream, sour cream, butter, cheese, ice cream, and even yogurt can increase acid in the stomach and slow down motility, which means that regurgitated material remains in the esophagus longer, burning the delicate tissues.

TOMATOES

Tomatoes have a high acid content. They can irritate the lining of the esophagus and aggravate heartburn. This includes raw tomatoes in a salad, tomato sauce on pizza and pasta, catsup, and tomato juice.

ONIONS

Onions are another vegetable with a high acid content that can make your heartburn worse. When people say that onions "repeat" on them, what they are really saying is that onions cause acid reflux for them.

SPICES (PEPPER, CURRY, CHILI POWDER, AND SO ON)

These spices and the foods they are found in can be potent triggers of both heartburn and other symptoms of GERD.

NUTS

Nuts are fatty, and as with other fatty foods, they relax the LES, allowing some of the content of the stomach to flow backward into the esophagus.

CARBONATED BEVERAGES

The carbonation in soft drinks also relaxes the LES. Many people with heartburn and other symptoms of GERD are surprised when the carbonation makes them belch and they quickly experience a bitter taste in their mouths. It is because of the refluxed material from their stomach that has seeped in through the LES.

ALCOHOL

Alcohol in any form—beer, wine (especially red), and hard liquor—can worsen heartburn and other symptoms of GERD because alcohol tends to relax the LES. Alcohol also increases the amount of acid in the stomach, so it's a double whammy.

So What Can You Eat?

You may look at the list of possible foods to avoid and think, "There's nothing left for me to eat but bread and cheese. Whoops, no cheese because it's fatty and it's also a dairy product." But don't stop eating any food until you know for sure that it's a trigger for you. Chances are you probably can eat much of what is on the above list. It's possible that french fries, fried chicken, and chocolate cream pie may give you heartburn, but you can eat hot tamales, peppers, and chili without a care.

You'll have to work by trial and error (and with your physician) to figure out what triggers heartburn and other symptoms of GERD for you. *Never omit an entire food group without your doctor's permission.* There may be just one or two of those foods you should ignore. Keep a "GERD detection diary" to learn which food and drink give you trouble.

Keep a Detection Diary

The best way to determine what foods create heartburn and other symptoms of GERD for you is to keep a detection diary. Most of us don't have total recall and we tend to forget what we ate the day before, let alone what was a trigger for us a week ago when we sit down to eat it again.

For one week, write down *everything* you eat. Mark the time of the day when you ate the food, when you experienced heartburn or other symptoms, and what else was going on in your life at that time. This last is important. Your mind and emotions do affect your body. Your stomach certainly isn't an isolated part of you; it's a center of activity. When you're tired, anxious, or stressed, your stomach and the rest of your digestive system is affected as well.

Be conscientious and keep the detection diary for one week. Put some blank forms in your purse or pocket so you don't forget to list foods you eat away from home. But be patient. This isn't an exact science like being weighed or having your blood pressure taken. There's no neat computer printout that says, "Eat this!" or "Don't eat this!" You're going to have to figure it out for yourself by doing a little detective work.

After at least a week—though longer is better—spread out all the pages and arrange and rearrange them to see if you detect a pattern. If you notice more heartburn and reflux when you've had a fast-food burger or ice cream or three

GERD Detection Diary

Food or beverage consumed:_____

Time eaten: _____ Symptoms:_____

Time symptoms experienced:_____

Medications taken:_____

Hours passed before lying down:_____

Other activity (such as exercise):_____

Hours after eating:_____

Stress factors while eating: ___hurried ___fatigued ___angry ___no more than usual

glasses of red wine, then you and your doctor will be able to modify your diet accordingly.

Write legibly, and if you use abbreviations, be sure you remember what they are. A week later you won't remember whether "Fat" meant "fatigued," "fatty meal," or "fruit and tea."

You can make lots of photocopies of the detection diary. The International Foundation for Functional Gastrointestinal Disorders (IFFGD) offers a one-week diary that serves the same purpose. To get one, call toll free 1-888-964-2001 or visit their Web site at www.IFFGD.org.

The Woolf Maxim

The English author Virginia Woolf had it right when she said, "One cannot think well, love well, sleep well, if one has not dined well." Eating is a part of socializing in our society. Don't think that just because you have gastroesophageal reflux disease you have to become a recluse and never go out to eat. Take the time to learn what triggers your discomfort, then work with your physician to create an eating plan that satisfies, lets you socialize, yet keeps you free from pain. This strategy may include other lifestyle modifications and it may also include medication.

Treating GERD is a team effort. Don't try to handle it alone.

Medications That May Be Effective

Keep a watch also on the faults of the patients, which often make them lie about the taking of things prescribed.

— HIPPOCRATES

THERE ARE numerous medications, both prescription and over-the-counter, as well as herbal preparations that can be used in treating gastroesophageal reflux disease and its various symptoms. Each type of drug works in its own way, and some of them are used in combination with others for greatest relief. If one type of medication doesn't help you, there are others that may. There is no "one pill cures all" for GERD; treatment and choice of drug therapy depend on each individual and his or her degree of symptoms along with other existing medical conditions. Even the dosage may differ from person to person, so don't be concerned if your physician prescribes a different dosage of the same medication a friend or coworker is taking.

Antacids

You're probably most familiar with the antacids such as Tums, Rolaids, Mylanta, and Maalox, medications that can be bought over-the-counter without a prescription. Antacids neutralize existing stomach acid and are usually effective in just minutes. You take them after you've eaten or begin to experience symptoms.

Unfortunately, the effect of antacids wears off in only an hour or so, as long as it takes for the drug to pass through the stomach, so antacids really are for fast, short-term relief. Experts say these familiar over-the-counter drugs are used regularly by at least a third of the population of the United States. But according to many concerned physicians, continual use of these medications may mask a more serious underlying problem. If you find yourself taking antacids for more than two weeks at a time, you should stop self-medicating and go to see your doctor. It's important to be examined by a physician to be sure you don't have esophagitis, Barrett's esophagus, or possible esophageal adenocarcinoma. Your doctor can also prescribe a stronger medical therapy for your GERD condition.

Antacids can reduce the effectiveness of a variety of other medications, such as antibiotics and heart and blood medications, so don't casually reach for an antacid if you're on these drugs for other conditions. Always check first with your physician.

H_2-Receptor Blockers

Another type of medication used to treat gastroesophageal reflux disease is the H_2 (histamine) receptor or acid blocker. This category includes Pepcid AC (famotidine), Tagamet HB (cimetidine), and Zantac 75 (ranitidine). Originally available only by prescription, the medications now can be purchased over-the-counter, although these OTC drugs are only half the strength of those obtained with a prescription.

These acid blockers prevent the release of stomach acid, so you should take them before you experience symptoms. Although it takes approximately an hour for the acid blocker to begin to work, the effects continue for nine to twelve hours.

As Tagamet can interact (by delaying breakdown by the liver) with theophylline you may be taking for asthma control, as well as with medications such as Dilantin and Coumadin, always check with your doctor before mixing medications.

Prokinetic Drugs

Prokinetic drugs increase peristalsis and make food move more rapidly through the digestive system, which helps to reduce the amount of time the acid stays in the esophagus. Reglan (metoclopramide) is an example of this type of medicine. It does have side effects, however, in a significant number of patients. Propulsid (cisapride) used to be prescribed for nighttime heartburn, but as it had serious side effects, including some fatalities, Propulsid is no longer available in the United States.

Proton Pump Inhibitors

These drugs, known as PPIs, include Prilosec (omeprazole), Prevacid (lansoprazole), Nexium (esomeprazole magnesium), Protonix (pantoprozole), and Aciphex (rabeprazole). They are considered to be the medication of choice in controlling GERD. PPIs have been in use in the United States for fifteen years (Prilosec in 1986, Prevacid in 1995, Aciphex in 1999, Protonix in 2000, and Nexium in 2001). Protonix is the only PPI that is also available in IV form, as well as in tablets to be taken orally.

The proton pump inhibitors work by actually preventing the formation of acid in the stomach. PPIs must be taken before meals to be most effective (usually before breakfast and dinner, if two doses are required). They proved not only to prevent heartburn, but also reduce symptoms of asthma, hoarseness, coughing, esophagitis, and many other of the atypical symptoms of GERD. In clinical use, proton pump inhibitors are said to be effective in controlling acid suppression in 80 to 100 percent of the cases. Doses may vary depending on the severity of your symptoms.

Some people experience relief from GERD symptoms throughout the day while they are taking Prilosec but still suffer from nocturnal reflux. Remember that PPIs need food to be activated. A recent study suggests that by adding an H_2 receptor at bedtime, these patients having breakthrough symptoms can be helped.[1]

All of these drugs, both OTC and prescription, may cause side effects depending on each individual's body makeup, coexisting medical conditions, and other medications being taken. Be sure your physician is aware of all medications you are using, including over-the-counter drugs, herbal preparations, anti-inflammatory drugs, aspirin, asthma medications, cortisone, or arthritis drugs.

As effective as many of these medications are in helping to alleviate the problems of heartburn and other symptoms of GERD, they must be used in addition to the lifestyle modifications mentioned earlier.

When Should Surgery Become an Option?

An hour of pain
is as long as
a day of pleasure.

— ENGLISH PROVERB

I DIDN'T COME easily to the decision to have surgery," Sydney, a literary agent, confided to me, running her fingers through her hair. "I had lived with so much pain for so long—nine years of burning sensations in my chest, constant sore throats, laryngitis, and a chronic cough. I was tired of taking hundreds of pills that really didn't help much. My husband and I wanted to start a family, and I wanted to feel better before I got pregnant. When my gastroenterologist said, 'If you want to, we can explore surgery,' I felt as though I might have a chance for a normal life again. I didn't hesitate long before saying yes."

Try Lifestyle Changes and Medications First

First choice in treatment always should be to try to minimize the pain of gastroesophageal reflux disease through lifestyle changes and medication. Most patients will be able to control their symptoms through a firm adherence to the lifestyle changes mentioned earlier as well as through careful use of various medications now available, such as the H_2 blockers like Tagamet, Zantac, and Pepcid and the proton pump inhibitors such as Prilosec, Prevacid, Nexium, Protonix, and Aciphex.

Have Patience

It's important not to get discouraged if medication doesn't immediately relieve your discomfort or downright pain. Sometimes it takes a while—often three months or even longer—for your physician to adjust the medication through trial and error and discover the ideal dosage and medicine or combination of medications that specifically work for you. Each of us is unique, and "one pill fits all" doesn't work, especially when you're dealing with multiple symptoms of GERD. Sometimes it may be as simple as changing the time of day you take a medication, such as before breakfast and dinner rather than after. It may require increasing or decreasing the dosage or even substituting one drug for another. It also may have a great deal to do with your physical makeup and condition. If you're a small woman, for example, you probably metabolize medication differently from a large man. It's possible that you may be taking additional medications for other medical conditions that interact adversely with the drugs needed to help your GERD.

You can help your physician by keeping track of your reactions to every new medication or dosage by actually writing them down in a notebook. The human mind can have a selective memory, and it's easy to forget exactly when certain symptoms lessened or how long others remained.

How to Know if You're a Candidate for Surgery

Be honest in evaluating whether you've made the necessary lifestyle changes such as losing weight, stopping smoking and drinking alcohol, and so on, and really stuck to them. Have you tried all the medications yet still have chronic and severe symptoms, as Sydney did? Do you feel that you can't face the thought of having to take medication for GERD for the rest of your life? Is the expense of surgery less than the cost of medication for the rest of your life? If the answer to all of the above is a resounding yes, then surgery may become a consideration.

It's estimated that approximately 5 percent of people with GERD will eventually require surgery. And for many, it also makes economic sense. A 1997 study of "Lifetime costs of surgical versus medical treatment of severe gastroesophageal reflux in Finland" concluded that ". . . antireflux surgery for GERD is cheaper than lifetime treatment with proton pump inhibitors."[2] Many others have come to the same realization.

Who is a good candidate for surgery? According to Donald van der Peet, a gastroesophageal surgeon at University Hospital Rotterdam in The Netherlands, "Any patient with GERD, whenever conservative measures fail (such as adverse effects of medication, perspective of life-long drug dependency, etc.), when GERD is objectively proven through manometry, 24-hour pH-metry, and so on, who respects the limitations of an anti-reflux procedure (including possible complications, etc.) is a potential candidate." Whereas van der Peet says he has no upward age limitation for surgery, he says that in his country "no gastroenterologist will refer a patient older than 75 years for this kind of surgery."

In material given to his prospective patients, Garth H. Ballantyne, M.D., chief of the Division of Laparoscopic Surgery, St. Luke's–Roosevelt Hospital Center in New York, stresses that, "Surgery is only recommended to patients with both a defective lower esophageal sphincter and a correlation between acid reflux and the onset of symptoms." According to Ballantyne and many other surgeons, fundoplication (the type of surgery) achieves excellent results in 90 to 95 percent of "carefully selected" patients. The "carefully selected" requirement seems to be extremely important.

In an article in *The American Journal of Gastroenterology*, Philip O. Katz, M.D., Vice Chairman of Medicine and Chief of Gastroenterology at Philadelphia's The Graduate Hospital, lists what he considers to be indications for surgery. According to Katz, "Antireflux surgery should be considered for the treatment of patients with objectively documented, relatively severe GERD, including patients with erosive esophagitis, stricture, and Barrett's esophagus, and for those without severe mucosal injury who require continuous high-dose PPIs for long-term symptom relief. Patients with atypical or respiratory symptoms who respond well to intensive medical treatment should be considered. The option of antireflux surgery should be given to all patients who require long-term aggressive medical therapy, particularly if escalating doses of PPIs are needed to control symptoms. Antireflux surgery may be the preferred option for patients less than 50 years of age, for those whose medications are a financial burden, for those who are noncompliant with their drug regimen, and for those who prefer a single intervention to long-term drug treatment."[3]

Being younger than fifty may be preferred, but it is not a rule. Patients over seventy-five have been operated on successfully. (So have infants and children, though that is uncommon.)

You may not be a candidate for surgery if you have specific other coexisting medical conditions, if you haven't responded to treatment with proton pump inhibitors, or if you have some of the atypical symptoms of GERD such as chest pain. Some surgeons hesitate to perform fundoplication on patients who have had previous abdominal surgery that may have created scarring. The patient selection process obviously is very important to the success of this procedure.

What Is the Surgery?

The most common surgery to repair the lower esophageal sphincter is called Nissen fundoplication, introduced by Rudolf Nissen, a German surgeon, in the 1950s. It involves wrapping the upper portion of the stomach around the lower part of the esophagus to create a new and tighter lower esophageal sphincter valve. This prevents the stomach acid from refluxing into the esophagus as it did before.

Before 1991, surgery for GERD, called open Nissen fundoplication, required the surgeon to make a six- to ten-inch incision in the patient's abdomen. Recovery was slow and painful, often requiring a long stay in the hospital of a week or more and taking as much as six to eight weeks to fully recover.

But since the use of laparoscopic surgery beginning in the late 1980s for gallbladder surgery, surgical repair for GERD using the laparoscopic Nissen fundoplication (LNF) procedure has become far easier for both the patient and the surgeon. At present, the surgery most commonly being done to reduce reflux is performed with a laparoscope. It's now a minimally invasive procedure. The average operating time runs between two and four hours, with some being done in ninety minutes. Most studies on the use of LNF with GERD agree that the cure rate of symptoms of heartburn, regurgitation, and pain when swallowing is more than 90 percent.

How Laparoscopic Nissen Fundoplication Surgery Is Performed

A laparoscope is a tiny tube with a miniature video camera at one end. With the patient under anesthesia, the abdomen is inflated with gas to make it an open hollow space. Five half-inch to quarter-inch incisions are made in the upper part of the patient's stomach. The laparoscope is then inserted into one of the holes, and it transmits highly magnified images of the area to a video screen. The surgeon watches the screen as he or she operates using instruments and retractors that have been placed in the other tiny openings.

Healing after laparoscopic Nissen fundoplication is speedy because there is no deep major incision. Patients experience less pain so they require less medication with its accompanying side effects, They have fewer complications, less scarring, and usually a shorter hospital stay, which lowers the risk of hospital-acquired infections. They also tend to return to work faster. According to Mark Pleatman, a surgeon in Rochester, Michigan, "Patients are up and walking by the next day."

Although the average hospital stay following an LNF is two to three days, many patients go home the day after the surgery.

According to Patrick Reardon, a surgeon at Baylor College of Medicine and The Methodist Hospital in Houston, "They [patients] can usually return to work within a few days and resume all activities after just one week."

A Swedish study compared the costs between the open and laparoscopic surgeries for GERD. They found that the laparoscopic group required a postoperative sick leave of only 9.9 days, compared to 29.9 days for patients undergoing the more extensive open surgery, and it also had a shorter period of rehabilitation. Although the actual cost of laparoscopic surgery is higher, the added expense of longer hospital stays required for the open fundoplication along with outpatient visits and other medical costs were almost twice as much with the open surgery.[4]

Surgical Risks and Side Effects

Because LNF is a fairly new procedure, there is little research compiled so far as to the extreme long-term benefits of this type of surgery, although according to surgeon Mark A. Pleatman, "90 percent of patients followed for as long as ten years are satisfied with the results." Most research studies confirm that the vast majority of those who had LNF are pleased with the results (even if they had some residual effects from the surgery) and would recommend the procedure to friends who fit the surgical profile.

But all surgical procedures, even laparoscopic ones, which for some reason seem "simpler" to many of us, carry a number of risks that you must be aware of before consenting to surgery. Even in the hands of a skilled surgeon there can be bleeding, perforation of nearby tissue, a danger of infection, and the possibility of a blood clot being dislodged.

Some people may experience a number of side effects, most of which are temporary, including some bloating (due to the inability to burp), difficulty swallowing due to the swelling of the tissues of the esophagus, the inability to vomit, and some discomfort or actual pain. While the incidence of postoperative dysphagia (difficulty swallowing) varies greatly, in most cases it is temporary and clears up within a month or so. If the problem doesn't clear up, the esophagus can be dilated (stretched) to create more space for food to pass through.

It's estimated that 30–60 percent of patients may still require supplemental medication for their reflux after the surgery. And others may have surgical-related problems to deal with. Nevertheless, most surgeons are pleased with the outcome using LNF and mention few cases where the surgery needed to be repeated. Most patients, it is important to note, have few or no side effects whatsoever.

Selecting a Competent and Experienced Surgeon

Once you're considering having surgery, it's vital for you to take your time and to be very careful in selecting a surgeon. In addition to getting recommendations from your own physician, ask others in the medical field to suggest the names of potential surgeons. Be sure that any surgeon you consider has had a great deal of experience actually performing the laparoscopic Nissen fundoplication, not just other laparoscopic surgeries. Experts suggest that a properly trained surgeon has performed (not just observed) thirty to fifty of these procedures.

If you can't find a surgeon who is experienced in performing laparoscopic Nissen fundoplication in your area, be willing to go to a major medical center where you can find these experienced surgeons. The success of LNF surgical therapy depends greatly upon the experience and expertise of your surgeon.

Your particular insurance plan may limit your choices of a surgeon, but never select a surgeon you don't feel comfortable with just because he or she is on your insurance plan. There are others.

Meeting with Your Surgeon

When you meet face-to-face with the surgeon, be prepared to ask a number of questions.[5]

- How many of this type of operation have you performed? (Observing the surgery is not the same as actually doing it.)

- What were the outcomes?

- Who will handle the anesthesia? (If you or a blood relative has had difficulty during a surgical procedure with anesthesia, be sure to tell the surgeon.)

- What complications or potential problems might I expect?

- Will you describe the procedure to me? (Many enlightened surgeons have booklets or videotapes for their prospective patients.)

- What should I expect when I wake up?

- How long should my recovery be? (When can you go back to work, eat normally, drive, resume sexual relations, not have discomfort, etc.?)

- What is your philosophy about pain control? (Surgeons vary in their thoughts about pain control. One end of the spectrum may feel that a little pain doesn't hurt you, while those at the other end don't want you to feel any pain at all and may oversedate you. Try for a physician whose philosophy toward pain control is somewhere in the middle.)

- What do you charge? If your insurance won't cover this type of surgery, discuss a plan for how you will be able to pay for it. Remember that you'll also be billed by the hospital, the anesthesiologist, and other specialists who take part in your care.

Tell your surgeon about any other existing medical conditions you may have that might affect you during or after the surgery. (Don't expect the physician to read your mind and never lie about alcohol usage or use of illegal drugs.)

The same holds true when you meet with your anesthesiologist. Be sure to tell this physician all the medications you're taking, including herbal and over-the-counter products, and if you smoke, drink alcohol, or use illegal drugs. According to Charles H. McLeskey, M.D., chair of anesthesiology and director of perioperative services at Scott &

White Hospital of Texas A&M University, "Millions of people are taking many herbal medications and we don't know enough about these products, their effects and interactions. Some herbals can interact with anesthetics and have adverse effects, while others pose potential risks regardless of their interaction with anesthesia." Some herbal supplements may act as a blood thinner and can inhibit blood clotting, which would cause excessive blood loss during surgery. Others may cause relaxation, which could have an additive effect when combined with the sedatives anesthesiologists often give patients before and during surgery. Many anesthesiologists recommend that their patients stop taking herbal medications two to three weeks before surgery.[6]

There are several free brochures you can get to help you learn more about an upcoming elective surgical procedure.

When You Need an Operation

A series of four public information brochures: "Who Should Do Your Operation?," "What Should Your Operation Cost?," "Giving Informed Consent," and "Should You Seek Consultation (Second Opinion)?"

> *The American College of Surgeons*
> *55 East Erie Street*
> *Chicago, IL 60611*

What You Should Know About Anesthesia

> *The American Society of Anesthesiologists*
> *520 North Northwest Highway*
> *Park Ridge, IL 60068*
> *847-825-5586*

or

> *The American Association of Nurse Anesthetists*
> *222 South Prospect Avenue*

Park Ridge, IL 60068
847-692-7050

Sydney's Story

Remember Sydney, the woman I mentioned at the beginning of this section? She did decide to have the LNF surgery when lifestyle changes and various prescription drugs failed to ease her reflux. She agreed to share her experiences to give you a sneak preview of what really happened before and after the surgery. (She was asleep during the surgery, of course!)

Remember, however, that just as no two individuals are alike, no two operations are exactly alike. The surgeon's experience, the patient's other coexisting physical and mental conditions, and various symptoms of the reflux disease itself make each case unique. Nevertheless, this story will tell you how one woman perceived laparoscopic Nissen fundoplication surgery.

"I was thirty-four when I had my surgery," Sydney said. "I was fortunate in that I live in New York City where there are many qualified surgeons, but if there aren't any in your community, don't be afraid to go to the next larger town where you can find a surgeon experienced in performing LNS.

"My primary physician had a brochure from one particular doctor that was crammed with information. This doctor also had a Web site that was quite specific in details. The surgeon was a pioneer in fundoplication surgery and at the time of my surgery had done more than 1,000 with a 96 percent rate. His secret is that he picks only excellent candidates and has very high criteria. I think it's important for anyone to ask a surgeon, 'What is your success rate?' and 'What are your criteria for a surgical candidate?'

"The day before the surgery I went in for pre-admitting and testing and got a copy of the hospital's Patient's Bill of Rights. I was told to fast after eight or nine o'clock that night.

I was afraid I'd have trouble sleeping. One of my business associates, a neuropsychiatrist, gave me a pep talk that helped a great deal. He said I should visualize burying all my worries about the surgery in the ground. Then I should visualize a positive outcome from the operation. I did and had no trouble sleeping.

"The next morning I went into the hospital. The surgeon's assistants asked me about any possible drug allergies, which is very important when you're having an anesthetic for any type of procedure. It's especially vital with digestive surgery as they don't want you to have a bad reaction to a medication, vomit, and rip out your stitches. As one of the medications I'd be taking could make me nauseated, they also gave me an antiemetic so I wouldn't get sick to my stomach. The assistants went over all the details of the surgery so I would know exactly what to expect.

"In between these interviews, I again used visualization to help me detach from the hustle and bustle of the waiting room. This visualizing helped me to remain calm when it was time for me to change into a gown and walk into the operating room, and I highly recommend trying it. (I did, however, also clutch my referral from the insurance company to make sure everyone knew that my insurance company had agreed to pay for the surgery.) Once I was on the table, they gave me something to make me relax, and that's the last I remember until the surgery was over.

"I was the last person that day to leave the recovery room as it took me a while to wake up. My throat was sore from the breathing tube they had put down my throat during the surgery. They also hadn't told me that I would have a catheter in my bladder to drain off urine. I had something like a kid's water wings on my legs that inflated and deflated, to help prevent blood clots. My main discomfort at that point was extreme dehydration, and they would give me only a few ice chips, then nothing more.

"They took me to my room where I would spend the night. I was getting pain medication as needed every four hours. This is not the time to be a martyr. Be aggressive and ask for the pain medication if you need it, because you heal faster when you're not in pain. I felt a dull aching in my midsection and had trouble sleeping, but by three in the morning, I felt better. I suddenly realized that it was the first time in years that I had spent a night without reflux pain. The healing part was amazing. Around seven that morning I felt that I had turned the corner and was anxious to go home.

"It's important to follow the doctor's instructions about eating. For the first week postop I drank liquids and ate soft foods like applesauce, Jell-O, chicken broth, ice cream, soft scrambled eggs, and mashed potatoes. I craved protein. I recommend that before you go in for surgery you shop ahead for plenty of soft foods, frozen fruit bars, and juices. I was told to avoid carbonated beverages.

"The surgeon had warned me to chew all foods very carefully. He said that 2 percent of the failure rate with this surgery is with people who try to eat steak and rip their internal stitches. I ate stuffing (carefully) at Thanksgiving a week later, missed only two weeks of work, and was downhill skiing in a month. Basically, I had only two real problems after the surgery. One was getting in and out of my bed, as it pulled on the stomach stitches. I actually strained mine that way and had to ice them down, so I suggest that others be very careful about turning their bodies. The other difficulty was really bad constipation. The doctor had warned me that it might be a problem, but I sort of lost track of how long it had continued. By the time I had gone more than a week without a bowel movement, I had gotten painfully impacted. Laxatives did nothing to help. I finally had to use an enema to clean me out.

"It's been one year since I had my fundoplication. I haven't had even one episode of reflux since then. Do I recommend the surgery? Absolutely, if you are a good candidate for it and you've found a surgeon experienced in doing it. With LNF you can say good-bye to reflux."

Alternative Medicine

The physician is only nature's assistant.

—GALEN

PERHAPS A better term than "alternative medicine" is "complementary medicine," because it's often used in conjunction with conventional Western medicine. Its use is rapidly increasing. According to the *Journal of the American Medical Association,* there were 386 million alternative therapy visits in 1990. By 1997, that figure had almost doubled to 629 million. Four of every ten people turn to unconventional treatments for their health concerns.

Because of this increased interest in and acceptance of alternative medicine, many insurance companies and HMOs are beginning to offer plans to compensate practitioners of this type of therapy. Even our often slow to react government understands people's growing interest in alternative medicine. In 1993, Congress created the Office of Alternative Medicine (OAM) at the prestigious National Institutes of Health. The OAM funds a number of studies, many of which relate to reducing stress and therefore the intensities of many diseases through such therapies as visualization, massage, biofeedback, and self-hypnosis.

At a Spiritual Healing conference in 1997 sponsored by Harvard Medical School, Dr. Herbert Benson, chief of the Division of Behavioral Medicine, Beth Israel Deaconess Medical School and president of the Mind/Body Institute, said, "Comprehensive health care today is like a three-legged stool. One leg is pharmaceuticals, another is surgery, and the third is what you are able to do for yourself. Mind/body medicine is strengthening that third leg, integrated with the other two legs."

What Is Alternative Medicine?

"The alternative medical traditions can be thought of as sharing a vitalistic orientation—that is, they all presuppose that there is a life force or vital energy involved in healing."[7] Many of these traditions include ancient and non-Western forms of treatment such as acupuncture, Ayurvedic medicine, herbal therapy, reflexology, guided imagery, yoga, and massage therapy, just to mention a few.

But you don't have to make an either-or decision. In many cases, Western medicine coexists side by side with alternative medicine. As Burton Goldberg writes in his book *Alternative Medicine: The Definitive Guide*, "The Chinese have a saying about the wisdom of 'walking on both feet,' which means using the best of Eastern and Western procedures."[8] Since 1993, even the National Institutes of Health has encouraged this type of cooperation between alternative and allopathic (Western) techniques and philosophies.

How Alternative Medicine Can Help Gastroesophageal Reflux Disease

In an earlier chapter you learned about many types of alternative therapies that could help you to alleviate some of the discomfort associated with gastroesophageal reflux disease, although you may not have realized that's what they were because they have become so accepted in today's world. But thirty to fifty years ago, most Western physicians would have scoffed if you said you were using yoga, tai chi, biofeedback, guided imagery, or massage therapy to help reduce stress. Lifestyle modifications such as eliminating certain foods, not smoking, reducing your consumption of alcohol, and avoiding caffeine products are all beneficial techniques for reducing the effects of GERD including some of the atypical symptoms. They are types of what's called alternative medicine too.

Those practicing alternative medication also prefer using

natural ingredients to heal, rather than synthetic or chemically formed drugs. One such herbal aid often recommended to aid digestion and reduce heartburn is chamomile tea, made from flowers of the same name. (Some people may be allergic to it.) The tea tends to relieve only heartburn, however. It is not able to cure GERD.

Warnings About Alternative Medicine

Andrew Weil, M.D., author of *Natural Health, Natural Medicine,* often prescribes herbal remedies to his patients. He warns, however, that these "medicinal plants are dilute forms of natural drugs. They are not foods or dietary supplements, and you should not take them casually or for no good reason, any more than you would take a pharmaceutical drug casually or for no good reason." In order to be an informed consumer, Weil stresses these facts:

- Loose herbs sold in bulk are probably worthless.

- Encapsulated, powdered herbs are also likely to be worthless.

- Herbal products may be contaminated or adulterated.

- Standardized extracts of medicinal plants are the most reliable preparations.

- Tinctures and freeze-dried extracts of medicinal plants are also useful.

- Discontinue use of any herbal product to which you have an adverse reaction.

- Do not take herbal medicines unless you need them.

- Experiment with herbal remedies conscientiously.[9]

Keep an Open Mind

If you have not considered any of these alternative therapies, keep an open mind. It's important, of course, to remain aware that if something sounds too good to be true, it probably is, so be careful that you don't get taken in by charlatans who prey on people in pain. Although many people have received some relief from heartburn and other GERD symptoms by practicing some of the alternative therapies, you also need to take advantage of the allopathic techniques, including endoscopy, medication, and, perhaps, surgery.

Ask your physician for his or her opinion about alternative therapies. Remember that everyone is different, and something that helps a friend or relative may not work for you. Yet if you approach it with an open mind, you may find that a great deal of relief is often available by your taking control of the mind/body connection.

Don't make it an either-or decision. Let the best of each therapy work in combination to help you minimize the pain of GERD, while acting promptly and wisely to take those steps necessary to prevent Barrett's esophagus or esophageal adenocarcinoma from developing.

Potential New Treatments: The Stretta Procedure and the Endoscopic Suturing System

The results of early clinical studies indicate that two new treatments for gastroesophageal reflux disease may prove to be an attractive alternative to current medication and surgical options. One, the Stretta Procedure, developed by Conway Stuart Medical, in Sunnyvale, California, is presently being performed at eleven university sites around the United States on an outpatient basis.

A narrow, flexible tube, called a catheter, with needle

electrodes on a balloon is inserted into the patient's throat and down the esophagus. The balloon is inflated at the LES. Then the physician delivers precisely controlled radio frequency energy into the tissue. This creates coagulate tissue in the muscle of the lower esophageal sphincter. Cool water floods the surface tissue to keep it cool and protected throughout the procedure. As these small areas of tissue damage are absorbed over a period of a few weeks, they shrink, creating a tighter LES, which provides increased resistance to reflux of stomach contents into the esophagus.

The Stretta Procedure takes about forty minutes, and the patient is able to return to full activity the following day. The cost is estimated at about the same as a year's supply of medication and about 20 percent of the cost of surgery. At this writing, more than 100 patients ages nineteen to seventy-six have been treated.

In May 2000, the FDA approved the Stretta Procedure. In a study of forty-seven patients followed for six months after the procedure, 70 percent had quit taking all their heartburn medications. Nevertheless, because the procedure is so new, long-term results are still unknown.

Another new form of treatment just approved by the FDA is the Endoscopic Suturing System, developed by a physician at the Royal College of London. With this procedure, the LES is sutured through endoscopy to tighten it by a tiny sewing machine–like device from within the esophagus. In a study that followed sixty-four patients for six months after the procedure, 67 percent had either no heartburn or only occasional episodes. As with the Stretta Procedure, the Endoscopic Suturing System is a recent innovation and gastroenterologists and others are anxious to learn its long-term effects.

Chapter Six

Myths Concerning Gastroesophageal Reflux Disease and Heartburn

Beware of false knowledge;
it is more dangerous than ignorance.

—GEORGE BERNARD SHAW

MYTHS ARE powerful. They not only perpetuate false information, they also prevent people from looking for facts. This is especially true in medicine, where desperate and sick people are willing to try almost anything in order to feel better. That's what makes those who are ill such easy prey in our society.

This chapter contains a number of myths or folklore that have sprung up like weeds concerning heartburn and other symptoms of gastroesophageal reflux disease. Some of these old wives' tales are funny. Others could be dangerous if they keep people from correctly preventing or treating their condition.

Listed below are some common misconceptions about heartburn and other symptoms of gastroesophageal reflux disease, followed by the facts as health care professionals understand them today.

MYTH: If you're taking over-the-counter antacids for heartburn, you don't need to see a doctor.
The truth: If you suffer from heartburn two or more times a week for two weeks, most health care professionals suggest you make an appointment to see your physician.

MYTH: Heartburn is inevitable, a normal part of "living the good life."
The truth: Heartburn is not inevitable, nor is it your fault. It is one of many other symptoms of gastroesophageal reflux disease (GERD), which is a medical condition that requires treatment so it doesn't become more serious. While certain foods, alcohol, being overweight, and other lifestyle conditions can aggravate your symptoms, these are triggers, not causes of heartburn or GERD.

MYTH: If you don't have heartburn, you couldn't have gastroesophageal reflux disease.
The truth: Heartburn is only one symptom of GERD and is not required for the diagnosis of GERD to be made. Sometimes you can have a very serious case of reflux, such as with Barrett's esophagus, a precancerous condition, and yet have no feeling of heartburn whatsoever.

MYTH: If you have chest pains, they probably are caused by heartburn, not heart trouble.
The truth: Although chest pain can be a symptom of atypical gastroesophageal reflux disease, it also could be a sign of heart trouble. Rather than guessing wrong, it's always wise to seek medical care immediately when experiencing chest pain.

MYTH: Drinking milk can cure an ulcer.

The truth: Milk is no longer considered the cure-all for ulcers as it was once thought to be. Actually, drinking milk can create additional problems for those with ulcers as well as gastroesophageal reflux disease. That's because the calcium in milk signals the stomach to create more acid.

MYTH: Certain foods trigger heartburn in everyone.

The truth: While there are certain foods that seem to trigger heartburn in a great many people, there are no definite foods that bother everyone with GERD. Whether or not a food bothers you can also depend on how much of it you eat and what else is going on in your life at the time. You can't divorce your emotions from your stomach.

MYTH: If you suffer from heartburn when you're pregnant, it means your baby will be born with lots of hair.

The truth: Although heartburn when you're pregnant may make you feel like tearing your hair, it doesn't mean your baby will be born looking like Samson.

MYTH: Infants and children don't get heartburn or GERD.

The truth: Infants—even newborns—and children do suffer from heartburn and GERD. While the majority of them eventually outgrow their GERD, some don't and carry it with them into adolescence and even adulthood.

MYTH: Heartburn can't hurt you.

The truth: Heartburn *can* hurt you. Untreated, it can become esophagitis, an erosive irritation of the esophagus. That condition can turn into Barrett's esophagus, a precancerous condition. Some people with Barrett's esophagus develop esophageal adenocarcinoma, a potentially fatal form of cancer.

MYTH: Smoking a cigarette helps relieve heartburn.

The truth: Actually, cigarette smoking contributes to heartburn. Heartburn occurs when the lower esophageal sphincter (LES), a muscle between the esophagus and stomach, relaxes, allowing the acidic contents of the stomach to splash back into the esophagus. Cigarette smoking can cause the LES to relax. Smoking also reduces the amount of saliva in your mouth. This means there is less saliva to wash acid out of the throat and esophagus, so it remains longer. By staying in these areas longer, more damage can be done to the delicate tissues of the throat and esophagus.

MYTH: Surgery is the only form of treatment for GERD.

The truth: Surgery is only one form of treatment for GERD. Lifestyle modifications and drug therapy are two other treatments. Surgery is usually considered only by those who have tried the other two modalities and not been satisfied with the results, who don't want to take medication for the rest of their life, or who don't want the expense of lifelong medication.

MYTH: Spicy foods and stress cause stomach ulcers.

The truth: According to the National Institutes of Health, almost all stomach ulcers are caused either by infection with a bacterium called *Helicobacter pylori* or by the use of pain medications such as aspirin, ibuprofen, or naproxen (Aleve). Spicy food and stress may aggravate ulcer symptoms in some people, but they do not cause ulcers.

Chapter Seven

Frequently Asked Questions About Heartburn and Gastroesophageal Reflux Disease

What is GERD? GERD stands for gastroesophageal reflux disease. It's a condition that occurs when the acid contents in the stomach reflux into the esophagus, irritating and burning the delicate tissue found there.

How many people have symptoms of GERD? More than 20 million people in the United States suffer from symptoms of heartburn daily. One hundred million have symptoms of heartburn at some time. There no doubt are far more than that because many people with GERD symptoms don't see a physician, assuming that it's "normal" to have these symptoms.

What causes GERD? GERD is caused by the lower esophageal sphincter (the valve between the lower part of the esophagus and the upper part of the stomach) not closing tightly and allowing stomach acid to reflux. It also can be caused by a delay in the stomach emptying so the partially digested material and acid sit in the stomach longer.

Is heartburn the same thing as GERD? Heartburn is just one of the many symptoms of GERD. There are many others, including regurgitation, coughing, hoarseness, chest pains, asthma, and difficulty swallowing.

What's the most common symptom of GERD? Heartburn probably is the most common symptom of GERD.

How do doctors know if you have GERD? Doctors can be fairly sure you have GERD after taking a careful history and doing a physical exam. If they prescribe medication that relieves your symptoms, it's fairly certain. But to be sure you have GERD and that there is no sign of Barrett's esophagus or cancer, an endoscopy (with biopsy) is the only definitive way to make the diagnosis.

What are possible complications of untreated GERD? If your GERD is untreated, you can develop esophagitis, ulcers, Barrett's esophagus, or even esophageal adenocarcinoma. Don't wait to get treatment.

Is GERD something you get from poor eating habits, or isn't it your fault? Although poor eating habits can trigger GERD, it is caused by a relaxed lower esophageal sphincter valve that doesn't close tightly, by delayed emptying in your stomach, or by a slow motility that keeps acid in your esophagus a long time. Other medical conditions and medications can contribute to these problems.

What are the possible side effects of long-term use of antacids? Long term use of calcium-based antacids can affect your kidneys, while those with bicarbonate can build up sodium in your system. The long-term use of antacids also can mask your true condition of GERD and because they seem to be controlling your symptoms of heartburn, create a delay in your getting the proper diagnosis of GERD.

When should people with symptoms of heartburn see a physician? If you've had heartburn for two weeks straight it's time to see your physician.

What type of doctor treats GERD? Your primary care physician can treat you for GERD, as can ENT specialists, obstetricians, pulmonary specialists, and others, although they all may send you to a gastroenterologist for various tests.

Can you have GERD if you don't have heartburn? Yes, heartburn is only one of many symptoms of GERD. If you suffer from reflux, chronic coughing, nocturnal asthma, chronic hoarseness, or chest pain, see your doctor.

Do medications ever make GERD worse? Many medications can make your symptoms of GERD worse. If you notice the symptoms intensifying shortly after taking a new medication, ask your doctor if you can try a different preparation. Never stop taking your medications without your doctor's permission.

Do children ever have GERD? Infants and children do have GERD. In babies, positioning is used to keep them upright during and after feedings. Formula may be thickened. Medications also are prescribed in certain cases.

Can being overweight increase your susceptibility to heartburn? Excessive weight can put pressure on the lower esophageal sphincter valve and prevent its closing tightly.

Can certain foods make GERD worse? Each person may find specific foods that make GERD worse. These foods might include coffee, alcohol, chocolate, citrus, tomatoes, and carbonated beverages, for example.

What treatment is available for GERD? The treatment used today to treat GERD includes lifestyle modifications, medications, and surgery.

What kind of surgery is used for GERD? A procedure known as laparoscopic Nissen fundoplication is the surgery of choice for GERD.

How do you know if you should consider surgery? If you have severe pain and discomfort, don't want to take medication for the rest of your life, and think the one-time charge of surgery is better than paying for medication for years, you might consider surgery.

Is hiatal hernia the same thing as GERD? A hiatal hernia is a portion of the stomach popping up through the diaphragm. It can intensify GERD but does not cause it. Everyone who suffers from Barrett's esophagus has a hiatal hernia, but you don't need to have one to have GERD.

Is GERD a genetic disease? Researchers at this time are unsure if GERD is a genetic disease. It does seem to run in families, however.

Do you ever get over GERD, or is it a chronic disease? In most cases, GERD is a chronic disease. It often is outgrown in infants and children, and pregnant women who suffer from GERD often seem cured once they deliver.

Does smoking hurt you if you have GERD? Yes, smoking lowers the pressure on the lower esophageal sphincter valve. It also reduces the amount of saliva that is meant to dilute any acid present in the esophagus.

Is it true that you can get cancer if you have GERD?
Yes, people with GERD are more likely to develop Barrett's esophagus, which is a precancerous condition. Once you develop esophageal adenocarcinoma, it is likely to be difficult to cure because it doesn't present with symptoms until it's been growing a while.

Where can I get accurate information about GERD?
There are two major organizations whose membership is primarily composed of gastroenterologists, experts in the field of digestive disorders. You can get information from both of them by writing to:

The American Gastroenterological Association
7910 Woodmont Avenue, 7th Floor
Bethesda, MD 30814
310-654-2055
www.gastro.org

The American College of Gastroenterology
4900 B. South 31 Street
Arlington, VA 22206-1656
1-800-478-2876
http://www.acg.gi.org

Conclusion

Knowledge itself is power.

—FRANCIS BACON

THERE ARE a few major points I'd like to leave with you concerning heartburn and gastroesophageal reflux disease.

- First and foremost, that heartburn is not merely a trivial condition to self-treat or ignore. If the symptoms persist for two weeks, you need to see a physician for proper assessment and treatment.

- You do not necessarily need to have heartburn to be suffering from GERD. Some of the other symptoms include regurgitation, hoarseness, chronic coughing, asthma (a large number of people with asthma also have GERD), chest pains, pain swallowing, and waking at night with a bitter taste in your mouth.

- GERD is a chronic disease in many people that will require continual therapy to prevent symptoms and complications.

- Ten to 15 percent of patients with chronic GERD symptoms seen by a gastroenterologist have Barrett's esophagus, a premalignant condition.

- You can have Barrett's esophagus without experiencing heartburn.

- Less than 1 percent each year of those known to have Barrett's esophagus will develop esophageal adenocarcinoma, a form of cancer that has a poor prognosis. While this may seem like a low percentage, it isn't if you're one of those in the 1 percent category.

- The rates of Barrett's esophagus and esophageal adenocarcinoma are increasing dramatically.

- Never ignore heartburn or the other symptoms of GERD. Your life can depend on it.

Fortunately, the public is becoming more aware of the dangers connected with heartburn and GERD. In 1999, The American College of Gastroenterology (ACG) conducted a National GERD Public Education program. More than 900,000 prospective patients responded to their TV announcements and received both educational information on heartburn as well as the names and addresses of ACG member physicians.

You can still get this information by contacting the American College of Gastroenterology at their toll free number, 1-800-HRTBURN.

What the Future Holds

Researchers and clinicians are concerned about the rapidly increasing incidence of both Barrett's esophagus and esophageal adenocarcinoma. While cost factors make it impossible to use endoscopy and biopsy with every patient, certainly those not responding to lifestyle modifications and medications need to be tested further to rule out complications, Barrett's esophagus, or cancer.

Greater Awareness on the Part of Physicians

According to Dr. Joel Richter, "Physicians are increasingly aware that GERD may have atypical presentations such that the patient may initially present to cardiologists, pulmonologists, ENT physicians, or even obstetricians."[1] These and other specialists are becoming better informed about the symptoms of GERD—typical and atypical—and are making the diagnosis more quickly, which means that you can begin treatment before the disease evolves into a more serious condition.

New Medications

New medications are being devised to treat symptoms of GERD. The dark side to this is that as the drugs become easily available to the general population, people may self-diagnose and treat themselves rather than see their physician.

New Treatments

Exciting new treatments such as photodynamic therapy (PDT) offer great promise in the treatment of Barrett's esophagus. Other therapies under investigation include using heat (thermal ablation) or ultrasonic devices to destroy precancerous tissue, and cryotherapy, which involves using liquid nitrogen. Dr. Bergein F. Overholt suggests that it's probably a combination of methods that will be used for greatest success.

Aging of the Population

As the population of the United States and other Western countries continues to age, it's probable that the incidence of GERD with its complications may increase as well.

Our Challeng

The goal for physicians, of course, is for each patient to obtain long-term relief of symptoms. But in order for our doctors to be able to achieve this ideal for each of us, we must become the first wave. We are the ones who must recognize our symptoms, regardless if they are typical or atypical, and make immediate contact with our physicians before the disease has a chance to intensify, becoming esophagitis, Barrett's esophagus, or esophageal adenocarcinoma.

The challenge is in our hands.

Glossary of Terms You Should Know

acid pump inhibitor. (*See* **proton pump inhibitors**).

acute. A disease or symptoms that appear quickly.

adenocarcinoma. A type of malignant epithelial cells.

alarm symptoms. Warnings of serious GERD, such as weight loss, anemia, atypical chest pain, difficulty swallowing, and gastrointestinal bleeding.

allopathic medicine. Using drugs and surgery to heal illnesses.

asthma. A respiratory disease that causes obstruction of the airways and results in wheezing, coughing, and excessive mucus production.

balloon photodynamic therapy. A procedure in which a special dye is inserted into the patient's vein. Two days later, a deflated balloon is inserted into the esophagus, then inflated. When a special type of laser probe is activated in the esophagus, the drug retained in these cells produces a chemical that kills abnormal cells.

barium swallow. A test in which the patient is given a barium sulfate drink as a contrast medium while having an X ray of the digestive system.

Barrett's esophagus. A change in the cells of the tissue lining the bottom of the esophagus so they more resemble those lining the walls of the stomach.

Bedge. A foam wedge device that slips under the bedsheet to keep a person's head at least six inches above the stomach in order to prevent reflux.

bloating. A feeling of being filled with gas.

bolus. A mass of partially chewed food mixed with saliva.

bougie. A tapered medical instrument that is used to dilate or stretch the wall of the esophagus.

cardialgia. *See* **heartburn.**

chronic. A disorder that continues over a long period of time.

chyme. The mass of semidigested food that passes from the stomach into the duodenum.

columnar or specialized intestinal metaplasia of the esophagus. Another name for Barrett's esophagus.

conscious sedation. A medication given during medical procedures that keeps the patient free of pain but able to respond to directions.

diaphragm. A large sheet of muscle that separates the stomach from the chest cavity.

diaphragmatic hiatus. The opening in the diaphragm through which the esophagus passes and attaches to the stomach.

dysphagia. Difficulty swallowing.

edema. Swelling due to accumulated fluid in the cells and tissues of the body.

endoscopy. Examination of a body cavity through the use of an instrument that permits the physician to view that cavity.

erosion. Damage to tissues.

erythema. Redness or inflammation of the skin.

esophageal dysmotility. Slowness of peristalsis in the esophagus.

esophageal manometry. A test in which a patient swallows a small rubber tube to measure pressure induced by the peristaltic movement.

esophagectomy. A surgical procedure in which a portion of the esophagus is removed.

esophagitis. Inflammation of the esophagus that can be due to regurgitation of stomach acid.

esophagus. The muscular tube through which food passes from the throat to the stomach. In adults it is about 10 inches long.

fundoplication. A surgical operation in which the top part of the stomach is wrapped around the lower end of the esophagus, thereby preventing reflux.

gastritis. Inflammation of the stomach lining.

gastroenterologist. A physician who specializes in treating disorders of the esophagus and digestive system.

gastroesophageal reflux disease (GERD). A disease in which the stomach acid flows backward into the esophagus, burning the delicate membranes there.

gastroparesis. Slow emptying of the stomach.

gerontologist. A physician specializing in diseases of and medicine for the elderly.

GI tract. The digestive tract from mouth to anus.

globus sensation. The feeling of having a lump in your throat.

gullet. Another term for **esophagus.**

heartburn. One of the symptoms of GERD; also the sensation experienced with various heart ailments. It's the feeling of a burning in the chest and throat, of indigestion or fullness in the chest. Also referred to as *pyrosis* or *condition of fire.*

hiatal hernia. A portion of the upper part of the stomach pushing up into the chest from the opening in the diaphragm. Also called *hiatus hernia.*

histamine (H_2) blockers. Medication that prevents stimulation of the acid-producing cells in the stomach.

laparoscope. A rigid instrument with built-in video camera for examining and operating inside the abdomen.

laryngitis. Inflammation of the larynx or "voice box" causing loss of speech or hoarseness.

larynx. The voice box, located at the top of the trachea.

lower esophageal sphincter (LES). The valve between the lower end of the esophagus and the top of the stomach. Its purpose is to keep the contents of the stomach from flowing backward into the esophagus.

metaplasia. Tissue change.

metastasis. The spread of a cancer cell or tumor to another part of the body.

mucosa. The membrane or lining of the body passages, such as in the stomach and esophagus.

mucous membrane. *See* **mucosa.**

nissen fundoplication. *See* **fundoplication.**

nocturnal asthma. Awakening with coughing, wheezing, choking, or hoarseness.

nosocomial infection. An infection picked up at the hospital.

occult bleeding. Hidden bleeding that you are not aware of.

odynophagia. Painful swallowing.

otolaryngologist. A physician, popularly known as an ENT, specializing in caring for people with diseases and disorders affecting the ear, respiratory and upper alimentary systems and related structures, and the head and neck in general.

pediatrician. A physician who specializes in the care of infants and children.

peristalsis. A wave-like movement of muscle in the esophagus, stomach, and intestines that moves along food and liquid.

pH probe study. Measurement of the acidity or alkalinity by one or more sensors included in a small plastic tube passed via the nose and into the esophagus and/or stomach.

pill esophagitis. Inflammation of the esophagus due to a pill getting stuck in the throat, usually due to not drinking enough water with the medication or by taking medication while lying down or leaning backward.

prokinetic agents. Drugs that stimulate gastrointestinal motility to facilitate faster esophageal or stomach emptying.

proton pump inhibitors. Medications used to stop formulation of acid in the stomach cell at the final step in acid production.

pulmonologist. A physician who specializes in the lungs.

pyrosis. *See* **heartburn.**

regurgitation. The backward movement of esophageal or stomach contents into the throat and mouth.

rheumatologist. A physician who specializes in disorders of bones, joints, and connective tissues.

scleroderma. A progressive disease causing a hardening and thickening of the skin and also affecting the smooth muscles of the body's organ systems.

silent reflux. Reflux that occurs without symptoms.

squamous cell carcinoma of the esophagus. Cancer of the squamous cells of the esophagus mucosal lining.

staging. Performing various tests to determine the extent of a cancer and whether it has spread to other parts of the body.

stomach. The hollow organ located below the esophagus that receives food and chemicals and begins churning and breaking up food articles.

stricture. A narrowing of a hollow organ of the body, such as the esophagus.

ulcer. A destruction of tissue in the esophagus, stomach, or intestine that extends completely through the first inside layer (mucosa) to the second layer (submucosa) or even deeper.

upper GI series. An X ray examination of esophagus, stomach, and duodenum using swallowed barium to outline these organs and their diseases.

xerostomia. Dry mouth.

Chapter One
1. *JAMA*, 276, no. 12 (September 25, 1996).

Chapter Two
1. Oliveria, Susan A., ScD, MPH, et al. "Heartburn Risk Factors, Knowledge, and Prevention Strategies: A Population-Based Survey of Individuals with Heartburn." *Archives of Internal Medicine* 159 (July 26, 1999): 1594.

2. Friedman, Meyer T., and Ray H. Rosenman. *Type A Behavior and Your Heart*. New York: Alfred A. Knopf, 1974, p. 67.

3. Chopra, Deepak. *Quantum Healing*. New York: Bantam Books, 1989, p. 14.

4. Shimberg, Elaine Fantle. *Depression: What Families Should Know*. New York: Ballantine Books, 1991, p. 111.

5. Clark, C. Scott, M.D., et al. "Gastroesophageal Reflux Induced by Exercise in Healthy Volunteers." *JAMA* 261, no. 24 (June 23/30, 1989): 3599.

6. Weil, Andrew, Dr. *Self-Healing,* December 1999, p. 2.

7. Quoted in Lee, Michelle. "Secret Stress Therapies." *Men's Health,* September 1999, p. 97.

8. Quoted in Hirt-Manheimer, Aron. "Overcoming Our Pain: The Life Lessons of Dr. Bernie S. Siegel." *Reform Judaism* 24, no. 4 (Summer 1996): 42.

9. Tierney, Lawrence M., Jr., Stephen J. McPhee, and Maxine A. Papadakis, eds. *Current Medical Diagnosis & Treatment.* 38th ed. Stamford, CT: Appleton & Lange, 1999, p. 1186.

10. Tolia, Vasundhara. "Gastroesophageal Reflux in Infants and Children." *Clinical Practice of Gastroenterology* 2 (1999): 1251.

11. Ghaem, M., et al. "The Sleep Patterns of Infants and Young Children with Gastro-oesophageal Reflux." *Journal of Paediatric Child Health* 34, no. 2 (April 1998): 160–63.

12. Barmby, Laura C. *Breastfeeding the Baby with Reflux.* Schaumburg, IL: La Leche League, 1999.

13. Balson, Boris M., et al. "Gastroesophageal Reflux Widespread in Refractory Pediatric Asthma." *Annals of Allergy, Asthma and Immunology* 81 (August 1998): 159–64.

14. Sontag, Stephen, M.D., "Eating Before Sleep May Promote Reflux." *Executive Health's Good Health Report* 34, no. 4 (January 1998): 7.

15. Lluch, Irene, M.D., et al., "Gastroesophageal Reflux in Diabetes Mellitus." *The American Journal of Gastroenterology* 94, no. 4 (1999): 919–24.

16. Shoenut, J. P., J. A. Wieler, and A. B. Micflikier. "The Extent and Pattern of Gastro-oesophageal Reflux in Patients with Scleroderma Oesophagus: The Effects of Low-Dose Omeprazole." *Aliment Pharmacology Therapy* 7 (1993): 509–13.

17. Hassall, Eric. "Co-Morbidities in Childhood Barrett's Esophagus." *Journal of Pediatric Gastro and Nutrition* 25, no. 3 (September 1997): 255–60.

18. Lichtenstein, D. R., S. Syngal, and M. M. Wolfe. "Nonsteroidal Antiinflammatory Drugs and the Gastrointestinal Tract: The Double-Edged Sword." *Arthritis Rheum* 38 (1995): 5–18.

19. Wolfe, M. M., M.D., et al. "Gastrointestinal Toxicity of Nonsteroidal Antiinflammatory Drugs." *New England Journal of Medicine* 340, no. 24 (June 17, 1999): 1888.

20. Graedon, Joe, and Teresa Graedon, Ph.D. *Dangerous Drug Interactions.* New York: St. Martin's Press, 1999, p. 20.

Chapter Three

1. Theodoropoulos, D. S., et al. "Gastroesophageal Reflux and Asthma: A Review of Pathogenesis, Diagnosis, and Therapy." *Allergy* 54 (1999): 651–61.

2. Balson, Boris M., et al, "Gastroesophageal Reflux Widespread in Refractory Pediatric Asthma." *Annals of Allergy, Asthma and Immunology* 81 (1998): 159–64.

3. Irwin, Richard S. "Silencing Chronic Cough." *Hospital Practice* (January 15, 1999): 54.

4. Koufman, J. A. "The Otolaryngolic Manifestations of Gastroesophageal Reflux Disease: A Clinical Investigation of 225 Patients Using Ambulatory pH Monitoring and an Experimental Investigation of the Role of Acid and Pepsin in the Development of Laryngeal Injury." *Laryngoscope* 101 (1991): 1–12.

5. Irwin, R. S., et al. "Chronic Cough Due to Gastroesophageal Reflux: Clinical, Diagnostic and Pathogenic Aspects." *Chest* 194 (1993): 1511–17.

6. Bartlett, D. W., D. F. Evans, and B. G. Smith, Dept. of Conservative Dentistry, UMDS, Guys Hospital, London. "The Relationship Between Gastroesophageal Reflux Disease and Dental Erosion." *Journal of Oral Rehabilitation* (1996).

7. Schroeder, Patrick L., M.D., et al. "Dental Erosion and Acid Reflux Disease." *Annals of Internal Medicine* 122, no. 11 (June 1, 1995): 813.

8. Reynolds, James C., M.D., et al. "Barrett's Esophagus: Reducing the Risk of Progression to Adenocarcinoma." *Gastroenterology Clinics of North America* 28, no. 4 (December 1999): 917.

9. Tierney, McPhee, and Papadakis, *Current Medical Diagnosis & Treatment,* 1999, p. 566.

10. Overholt, Bergein F., M.D. "Esophagology for Clinician: Pathophysiology, Diagnosis & Therapy." Lecture, University of South Florida College of Medicine, December 2, 1999.

11. Harras, A., et al., eds. "Cancer Rates and Risks." 4th ed. Washington, DC: Department of Health and Human Services, National Institutes of Health, 1996. NIH publication 96–691.

12. Lagergren, Jesper, et al. "Symptomatic Gastroesophageal Reflux as a Risk Factor for Esophageal Adenocarcinoma." *The New England Journal of Medicine* 340, no. 11 (March 18, 1999): 825–11.

13. O'Sullivan, G. C., et al. "Micrometasteses in Esophagogastric Cancer: High Detection Rate in Resected Rib Segments." *Gastroenterology* 116 (1999): 543–48.

Chapter Four
1. Adapted from Blau, Sheldon P., and Elaine Fantle Shimberg. *How to Get Out of the Hospital Alive.* New York: Macmillan, 1997, pp. 199–201.

Chapter Five
1. Peghini, P. L., P. O. Katz, and D. O. Castell. "Ranitidine Controls Nocturnal Gastric Acid Breakthrough on Omeprazole: A Controlled Study in Normal Subjects." *Gastroenterology* 115 (1998): 1335–39.

2. Viljakka, M., J. Nevalainen, and J. Isolauri. "Lifetime Costs of Surgical versus Medical Treatment of Severe

Gastro-oesophageal Reflux Disease in Finland." *Scandinavian Journal of Gastroenterology* 32, no. 8 (August 1997): 766–72.

3. Katz, Philip O. "Treatment of Gastroesophageal Reflux Disease: Use of Algorithms to Aid in Management." *American Journal of Gastroenterology* 94, no. 11 (supp. 1999).

4. Blomqvist, A. M. K., et al. "Laparoscopic or Open Fundoplication?" *Surgical Endoscopy* 12 (1998): 1209–12.

5. Adapted from Blau and Shimberg, *How to Get Out of the Hospital Alive,* pp. 143–47.

6. American Society of Anesthesiologists. Press release, October 11, 1999.

7. Collinge, William, M.P.H., Ph.D. *The American Holistic Health Association Complete Guide to Alternative Medicine.* New York: Warner Books, 1996, p. 309.

8. Goldberg, Burton. *Alternative Medicine: The Definitive Guide.* Tiburon, CA: Future Medicine Publishing, 1999, p. xxxvii.

9. Weil, Andrew, M.D., *Natural Health, Natural Medicine.* Boston: Houghton Mifflin, 1998, pp. 235–37.

Conclusion

1. Richter, J. E. "Extraesophageal Presentations of Gastroesophageal Reflux Disease." *Seminars Gastrointest. Dis.* 8 (1997): 75–89.

Suggested Reading

Benson, Herbert, M.D., with Miriam Klipper. *The Relaxation Response.* New York: Avon Books, 1975.

Benson, Herbert, M.D., with Marge Stark. *Timeless Healing: The Power and Biology of Belief.* New York: Scribner, 1996.

Blau, Sheldon P., M.D., and Elaine Fantle Shimberg. *How to Get Out of the Hospital Alive.* New York: Macmillan, 1997.

Castell, D. O., M.D., and J. E. Richter, M.D. *The Esophagus,* 3rd Edition, New York: Lippincott Raven, 1999.

Collinge, William, M.P.H., Ph.D. *The American Holistic Health Association Complete Guide to Alternative Medicine.* New York: Warner Books, 1996.

Cousins, Norman. *Anatomy of an Illness.* New York: Bantam, 1981.

Graedon, Joe, and Teresa Graedon, Ph.D. *Dangerous Drug Interactions.* New York: St. Martin's Press, 1999.

Janowitz, Henry D. *Good Foods for Bad Stomachs.* New York: Oxford Press, 1998.

Nuland, Sherwin B. *Wisdom of the Body.* New York: Knopf, 1997.

Peikin, Steven, M.D. *Gastrointestinal Health.* New York: HarperCollins, 1991.

Wolfe, M. Michael, M.D., and Thomas Neal. *Heartburn: Extinguishing the Fire Inside.* New York: Norton, 1997.

Wolfe, Sidney M., M.D., Larry D. Sasich, Pharm.D., M.P.H., Rose-Ellen Hope, R.Ph., and Public Citizens Health Research Group. *Worst Pills, Best Pills: A Consumer's Guide to Avoiding Drug-Induced Death or Illness.* New York: Pocket Books, 1999.

American Academy of Otolaryngologists–Head and Neck Surgery
    One Prince Street
    Alexandria, VA 22314
    For a free leaflet on swallowing, send a stamped, self-addressed, business-size envelope.

American Association of Nurse Anesthetists
    222 South Prospect Avenue
    Park Ridge, IL 60008
    847-692-7050
    Ask for their free booklet, "What You Should Know About Anesthesia."

American Cancer Society
    1-800-227-2345
    www.cancer.org

American College of Gastroenterology
    4900 B. South 31st Street
    Arlington, VA 22206
    1-800-HRTBURN (1-800-478-2876)
    http://www.acg.gi.org
    This organization has information that may be of interest to those suffering from heartburn and GERD.

American College of Surgeons
    55 East Erie Street
    Chicago, IL 60611
    Ask for their free booklet, "When You Need an Operation."

American Gastroenterological Association
    7910 Woodmont Avenue, 7th Floor
    Bethesda, MD 30814
    301-654-2055, ext. 650
    www.gastro.org

American Osteopathic Association
    142 East Ontario Street
    Chicago, IL 60611
    1-800-621-1773
    www.aoa_net.org

American Society of Anesthesiologists
    520 North Northwest Highway
    Park Ridge, IL 60068
    847-825-5586
    Ask for their free booklet, "What You Should Know About Anesthesia."

Bedge
    For information on Bedge, the polyester foam wedge that elevates the entire upper body to ensure an antireflux sleeping angle, call 1-800-525-4820.

The Biofeedback Certification Institute of America
> 10200 West 44th Avenue, Suite 310
> Wheat Ridge, CO 80033
> www.bcia.org.

Consumer Nutrition Hotline of the National Center for Nutrition & Dietetics
> 1-800-366-1655
> Monday–Friday, 9 A.M.–4 P.M. Central time

Cleveland Clinic Hospital
> Joel Richter, M.D.
> 9500 Euclid Avenue
> Cleveland, OH 44195
> 216-444-6536

Froedtert Memorial Lutheran Hospital
> Reza Shaker, M.D.
> Medical College of Wisconsin Dysphagia Institute
> Division of Gastroenterology and Hepatology
> 9200 West Wisconsin Avenue
> Milwaukee, WI 53226
> 414-456-6840
> Fax: 414-456-6215
> E-mail: rshaker@mcw.edu

Gastric Reflux Association for the Support of Parents/Babies (GRASP)
> Attn: Rochelle Wilson, National Co-ordinator
> 307 Hendersons Road
> Hoon Hay
> Christchurch, New Zealand
> 03-338-2794 or (New Zealand 0800-380-517)
> E-mail: grasp@clear.net.nz.

Graduate Hospital, Digestive Institute
Donald O. Castell, M.D.
Philip O. Katz, M.D.
1800 Lombard Street
Philadelphia, PA 19146
215-893-7450
Fax: 215-893-2472 ·

International Foundation for Functional Gastrointestinal Disorders
PO Box 170864
Milwaukee, WI 53217-8076
1-888-964-2001
www.IFFGD.org
Monday–Friday, 9:30 A.M.–6 P.M. Eastern time
*Will answer questions about GERD without charge.
For $25 you can become a member and receive quarterly
newsletters, several publications about dietary considera-
tions, and an overview of GERD.*

Johns Hopkins Hospital
William J. Ravich, M.D.
600 North Wolfe Street
Gastroenterology
Baltimore, MD 21287
410-614-1280
E-mail: wravich@welchlink.welch.jhu.edu

La Leche League International
847-519-7730
www.lalecheleague.org

The Mind/Body Institute
Division of Behavioral Medicine
New England Deaconess Hospital
1 Deaconess Road
Boston, MA 02215
617-632-9525

National Cancer Institute
>   1-800-422-6237
>   *Ask for booklet, "What You Need to Know About Cancer of the Esophagus." Staff can talk to you in either English or Spanish.*

National Digestive Diseases Information Clearinghouse
>   2 Information Way
>   Bethesda, MD 20892-3560
>   301-654-3810
>   Fax: 301-907-8906
>   http://www.niddk.nih.gov>
>   E-mail: nddic@info.niddk.nih.gov

The National Exchange Club Foundation
>   1-800-760-3413
>   www.preventabuse.com
>   E-mail: info@preventchildabuse.com

Northwestern University
>   Comprehensive Center for the Treatment of
>   Esophageal Disease
>   Peter J. Kahrilas, M.D.
>   Professor of Medicine
>   Division Chief Gastroenterology & Hepatology
>   675 N. St. Clair, Suite 17-250
>   Chicago, IL 60611
>   Coordinator: Pamela Graham, LPN, BS
>   312-503-4375
>   E-mail: pgraham@nmff.nwu.edu
>   *As the office line is often hard to get through, use E-mail for faster service.*

Office of Alternative Medicine
National Institutes of Health
9000 Rockville Pike
Bldg. 31, #5B-37
MS 2182
Bethesda, MD 20892
301-496-1712
Fax: 301-402-4741

Pediatric/Adolescent Gastroesophageal Reflux Association (PAGER)
PO Box 1153
Germantown, MD 20875-1153
Main office: 301-601-9541
West Coast office: 760-747-5001
http://www.reflux.org/
A nonprofit organization that provides information and support to parents, patients, and doctors.

Thompson Cancer Survival Center
Photodynamic Therapy
1915 White Avenue
Knoxville, TN 37916
865-541-1678

University of Southern California School of Medicine
Tom R. DeMeester, M.D.
Department of Surgery
1510 San Pablo Street, Suite 514
Los Angeles, CA 90033-4612
323-442-5922
Fax: 323-442-5872
E-mail: demeester@surgery.hsc.usc.edu

University of South Florida Joy McCann Culverhouse Center for Swallowing Disorders
      H. Worth Boyce, M.D., Director
      USF Medical Clinic
      12901 Bruce B. Downs Boulevard
      MDC Box 72
      Tampa, FL 33612

Vomiting Infants Support Association (VISA)
      Leonie Ford, Secretary
      PO Box 4105
      East Gosford
      New South Wales 2250
      Australia
      Offers education and support to parents of infants and children with gastric reflux.

Index